SACRED SPACE

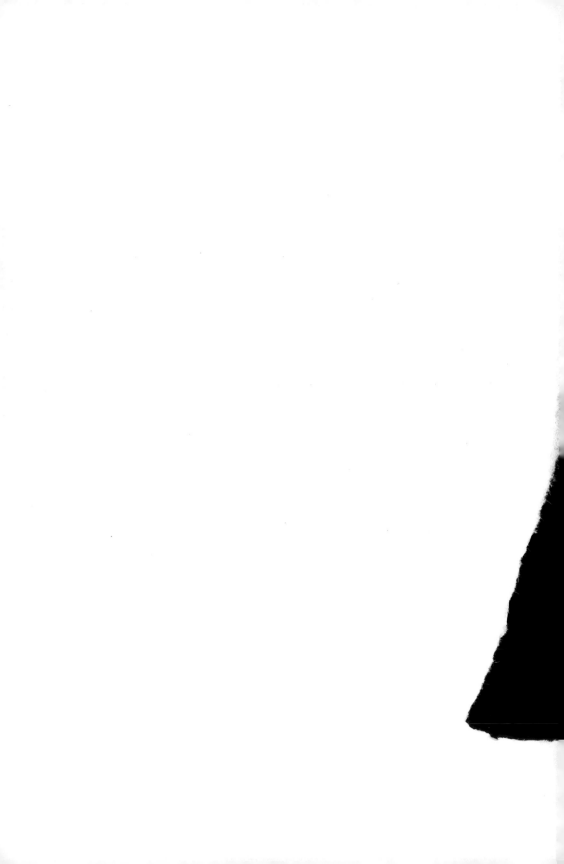

SACRED
SPACE

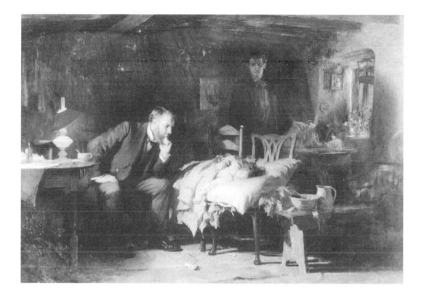

STORIES FROM

A LIFE IN MEDICINE

Clif Cleaveland, MD, MACP

AMERICAN COLLEGE OF PHYSICIANS
PHILADELPHIA, PENNSYLVANIA

A|C|P

Manager, Books Program: David Myers
Production Supervisor: Allan S. Kleinberg
Production Editor: Amy L. Cannon
Interior and Cover Designer: Kate Nichols
Dust Jacket and Title Page Painting: "The Doctor." Sir (Samuel) Luke Fildes (1843-1927).
Exhibited 1891. Tate Gallery, London. Courtesy of Tate Gallery, London/Art Resource, New York.

Publisher's Note—Pseudonyms are used for the people mentioned in *Sacred Space*, unless permission for use of real names has been granted.

Composition by Wendy Smith, American College of Physicians.

Printed in the United States of America by R.R. Donnelley, Harrisonburg, Virginia.

Library of Congress Cataloging in Publication Data
Cleaveland, Clif, 1936-   .
    Sacred space: stories from a life in medicine / Clif Cleaveland.
      p.   cm.
    ISBN 0-943126-64-9 (hard cover)
    1. Cleaveland, Clif, 1936-   . 2. Physicians—United States—Biography. I. Title.
    [DNLM: 1. Cleaveland, Clif, 1936-   . 2. Physicians—personal narratives. WZ 100 C623 1998]
R154.C345A3 1998
610'.92—dc21
[B]
DNLM/DLC   97-36741
for Library of Congress   CIP

Also Available from the American College of Physicians
Community-Based Teaching: A Guide to Developing Education Programs for
    Medical Students and Residents in the Practitioner's Office
Medical Meanings: A Glossary of Word Origins
On Being a Doctor
This is Our Work: The Legacy of Sir William Osler
Who Has Seen a Blood Sugar? Reflections on Medical Education

For ordering information contact:
Customer Service Center
American College of Physicians
Independence Mall West
Sixth Street at Race
Philadelphia, PA 19106-1572
215-351-2600 or 800-523-1546, extension 2600

To Ruzha Pfeffer Cleaveland,

my wife and my best friend

CONTENTS

CONTENTS

CONTENTS

FOREWORD

Toward the end of my first year at Johns Hopkins Medical School, we got the word that the admissions committee had admitted a new member to our class—a Rhodes scholar, no less—to begin in the fall. After a year of vying for position with some of the most competitive medical students on the planet, I was not happy to be faced with the challenge of a "Rhodesian." But when he actually appeared on the scene, hostility evaporated in the warmth and humor of Clif Cleaveland's unique personality.

Each of the stories in this book bears testimony to Clif's interest in people, his ability to be himself in many circumstances, and the empathy which allows him to see people for themselves and never as objects. My friendship with Clif began in the Hopkins pressure cooker, grew in the mellower atmosphere of Vanderbilt, and has only grown greater as the years have passed. One of our great annual pleasures is the Reading Retreat weekend for the Tennessee Chapter of the American College of Physicians, organized by Clif and held in the idyllic surroundings of Fall Creek Falls State Park. These events are redoubled in enjoyment by the presence of Clif's wife Ruzha, who contributes not only her own luminous personality but also her very accomplished poetry.

In reading Clif's book I was struck by two things. First, although we were at the same places at the same times and often had similar experiences, we took away rather different memories. For example, instead of seeing Hopkins as a paradise for the workaholic, my memories are of the meticulous approach to patient care informed by both a sound science and a warm compassion for the person, an approach exemplified by such teachers as Phil Tumulty. Also, because I was still single and Clif and Ruzha were starting their family, our views of the Hopkins scene were doubtless very different. Second, it is clear that physicians born in the 1930s who came of age in the '50s and '60s learned an amazing amount from African Americans. Coming from a background of ingrained racial prejudice and learning to care for all sorts and conditions of people is a sufficient education unto itself.

Clif has been, and is, a physician whom I would choose in a flash to take care of me and mine. He is a physician of great intellectual capacity, interest, and curiosity about his patients, but his greatest attributes are his abilities to see his patients as people and to allow them to see him as a person. As he is a great admirer of David Rogers, I am a great admirer of David's father, Carl Rogers, who taught that the three qualities of a true therapist (read healer) are being one's real self, having unconditional positive regard for others, and feeling empathy. I think that Clif's book illustrates that he possesses all three of these qualities, and he employs them in patient care in a sacred space. This space may just be that place where the doctor helps the patient find the meaning in the illness experience. We can imagine every patient as having a life story which is broken or interrupted by illness. Part of healing is in repair of the patient's narrative. In the case of death, the break is in the family's narrative, and part of our job is to help them heal the story of their family. Clif is a healer of persons and a healer of narratives.

O. *Thomas Feagin,* MD
Memphis, Tennessee

PREFACE

From my earliest days in medical school onward, close, continuous relationships with my patients have represented the highest privilege of clinical practice. I had assumed that this interaction was integral to the care of sick people. Indeed, as technology flourished, the private and individualized encounters with my patients remained intact and crucial to the processes of diagnosis and therapy. The initial decisions of how to proceed and how intensively to treat rest upon detailed knowledge of what my patient and his or her closest family and friends value. This information is especially crucial when the end of life is near.

The phenomenon of so-called managed health care threatens to undo this traditional physician-patient relationship. No one could argue that the cost of health care in the United States is out of control or that without fresh thinking medical expenditures would place intolerable pressures upon personal, business, and governmental budgets. While some managed care enterprises have made sustained commitments to upholding quality, many other enterprises have placed their emphasis upon protocols that encourage cost reduction and speedy interaction over all else.

Employers naturally seek the least-costly health plans for their personnel. For my colleagues and me this has resulted in the abrupt shift of long-term patients from one physician to another at yearly intervals. Some health plans encourage the use of nonphysician "extenders" for such work as interviewing patients and treating less complex illnesses. In tightly capitated health plans in which the physician receives a pre-paid fixed budget for the care of patients, there are subtle pressures for avoiding patients with incurable or complex illnesses.

Increasingly, I deal with anonymous voices at toll-free numbers to determine what procedures and consultations can be approved for my patients. Sometimes these judgments are simply wrong-headed and unjust. In Tennessee the most exasperating example of telephonic oversight of medical care rests with behavioral health organizations. Their protocols require that I give to a patient who may be depressed a toll-free number. The patient then can be interviewed via telephone so that the interviewer can determine what medication or referral may be authorized.

My physician colleagues and I cherish and respect personal, on-going, confidential dealings with our patients. Intonations of speech and facial expressions tell what lies beyond our patients' descriptions of their symptoms and fears. Our styles of listening, explaining, and comforting must be carefully tailored to the complex needs of each individual patient.

I find myself in the midst of a revolution in health care in America. As traditional values and protocols for medical practice have been called into question, I realize anew the precious nature of the stories that my patients and teachers have entrusted to me. For me, these stories represent the very essence of medical care.

ACKNOWLEDGMENTS

I am grateful to the patients and their families who have shared their stories and their trusts with me from medical school onward. Their stories continue to inform and inspire me.

The staff of the Tate Gallery generously taught me about "The Doctor" during a visit to the museum. The Tate Gallery has permitted reproduction of this painting for this volume.

Maria Mitchell expertly and patiently typed the manuscript in its various stages. My nurse, Jane Plumlee, kept my clinical schedule under control while I wrote. Dr. Janice L. Willms of Missoula, Montana, Dr. Henry Schneiderman of West Hartford, Connecticut, my medical partner, Dr. Anne Barron, and my daughter-in-law, Sarah Cleaveland, provided sensitive and valuable critiques of the manuscript. My wife, Ruzha, provided invaluable editorial advice throughout.

David Myers and Mary Ruff of the Books Division of the American College of Physicians have guided this project with great patience from the outset.

INTRODUCTION
DEFINING THE SPACE

No image of medicine speaks to me more powerfully than "The Doctor," painted by the famed British social realist, Samuel Luke Fildes. The $8' \times 5'$ canvas hangs in London's Tate Gallery, where it has been housed since the founding of that magnificent museum in 1890. Postage stamps, commemorative prints, and porcelain objects have popularized this masterpiece to the extent that its powerful message may be overlooked.

The scene is familiar. A life hangs in delicate balance. At the bedside of the wan, curly haired child sits a physician, whose eyes and attention are riveted upon his young patient. His bearded countenance conveys both knowledge and deep concern. He contemplates the therapeutic options: What can yet be done to restore health to the terribly ill child stretched out before him? He senses the ebbing of the child's life. We sense that he has sat by this bedside for the entire night.

The child, boy or girl we cannot tell, is comatose or in a sleep of exhaustion. The left arm hangs flaccidly over the edge of a large pillow placed under the child's head. Heavy, rough covers have been partially pulled back, suggesting earlier chills and rigors. This is illness at its most grave.

Beyond the reach of the oil lamp the exhausted mother sits with her head buried in arms folded upon a tabletop. Her husband stands behind her chair, resting his left hand upon her shoulder. His face tells us of past sorrows and hard work. He tries to provide quiet strength for his spent, grieving wife.

The sickroom is modest. Two chairs pulled together form the child's cot. A pitcher and bowl rest upon a bench or seat at his head. A wrinkled rug covers a portion of the wooden floor. Overhead, a rough beam supports the low ceiling. This might be the interior in the village or country cottage of a laborer or farmer. Possibly, we are inside the London apartment of a carpenter or tradesman.

From the doctor's dress, the lamp, and the surroundings we place this tableau in the 19th century. Given that approximate time, the child might suffer from any of a host of childhood scourges. From Austin Flint's *Principles and Practice of Medicine* (1868), the doctor might have read:

> A pathological condition of much interest and importance has heretofore, and is still called pyaemia or purulent infection of the blood; called also pyogenic fever, pus-blood or purulent infection of the blood ... [T]he existence of the affection clinically known as pyaemia is to be determined during life by the occurrence of chills, rapidity and feebleness of the pulse, prostration, etc. ... [A] fatal termination in cases of so-called pyaemia is due to the destructive changes of the blood and the secondary affections ... [O]bjects of treatment, in general terms, are palliation of symptoms and support of the powers of life. Sustaining measures are especially indicated, the aim being to prolong life until the processes of restoration are completed.

From the same text the physician would derive a list of other possible diagnoses and treatments. If pneumonitis were present, tablespoons of brandy might be helpful as would "antimonial preparations."

> Blisters should not be employed. ... It is questionable whether blood letting be ever advisable in young children, even when the diagnosis is clear in the first stage of the disease.

Advanced tuberculosis would certainly be a possibility as would "cholera infantum," a severe, acute gastroenteritis. Flint further notes,

"Children of the poorer classes, in insalubrious situations, living in crowded dwellings, are more likely to be affected." Cerebrospinal meningitis, typhoid fever, and scarlet fever were prevalent among children of that day as well, and often were fatal.

Sir Luke Fildes brought together all of these elements in his deceptively straightforward canvas. I learned of the artist's inspiration from a guide at the Tate Gallery and from materials subsequently mailed to me by that gracious institution. Fildes' infant son died on Christmas morning 1877. The painting, completed 13 years later, commemorates the parents' deep regard for the physician who ministered to their child.

My first viewing of "The Doctor" followed years of clinical practice in a variety of settings. I stood before the painting for a long time during an afternoon of few visitors. I purchased a large print from the museum store, and this hangs opposite my desk where I can see it daily. Fildes defines a sacred space, or circle of caring, whose center is a terribly sick or injured fellow mortal. The caregiver, in this case a physician, and the beloved ones occupy the space and perhaps even protect it against intrusion. The space speaks of caring, of quiet, of compassion. Grief, exhaustion, fear, and even confusion are there as well. There is candor and inquiry, but overarching all are love and respect for human life.

In our day this sacred space may be in varied settings: an intensive care unit, a hospice or nursing home, an emergency room, and less often the patient's home.

Rather than a single doctor, a team of physicians, nurses, and technicians may provide professional care. The space may be stretched by limiting loved ones to hallways or distant waiting rooms. Irrespective of the setting and its accompanying noise and technologic intrusions, the space is imbued with the same characteristics so poignantly captured by Luke Fildes.

Issues of race, gender, religious creed, or economic circumstance should in no way lessen the care given in this space. Profit motives and bureaucratic regulation are alien to it. Scientific advances have brought healing to many situations that would have had fatal outcome a century ago. But illness always requires affectionate concern.

Here follow true stories that taught me of this sacred space.

LaGRANGE

1936~1950

I cost my parents thirty-seven dollars and fifty cents, that being the charge by the hospital of LaGrange, Georgia, for labor and delivery plus several days of room and board for my mother and me. A fractured clavicle and dented skull attested to the difficulty of pulling, by high forceps, a large baby from a small woman. The depression in my skull remains to this day.

My first focused and dated memory of childhood springs from a second birth, four years later in 1940, when my sister was born in less complicated fashion. I was allowed to ride home in the ambulance that carried my mother and new sibling.

The town of my first years straddled U.S. Highway 29 from Atlanta just before the road crossed the state line into Alabama. At the top of LaGrange's caste system were mill owners and their senior administrators. Families of merchants and salesmen occupied the next small niche, while the majority of families worked in the mills and struggled to get by. Mired deep at the bottom of this social and economic scale were the second, third, and fourth generations of descendants of African slaves.

The Marquis de Lafayette stopped there once, commenting that the area reminded him of his French estate "LaGrange," hence the name for my hometown. When Union troops pushed south from Atlanta, a fiercely determined group of local women confronted them on the road outside the town and dissuaded the soldiers from torching their community. Many antebellum homes remain as monuments to their bravery.

During my childhood, Court Square sat empty. The courthouse that held my birth certificate was burned by a religious sect whose members had been arrested for selling pamphlets without a license. In that square, on Saturday mornings, rival, raspy-voiced evangelists gathered to boom their messages through giant loudspeakers mounted atop their Hudsons and Terraplanes.

At the Court Square Pharmacy, a nickel purchased a scoop of vanilla ice cream topped with chocolate syrup, whipped cream, and a cherry. The shelves of that apothecary were lined with patent medicines, many of which depicted a mustached "doctor" on the label. One remains in my possession: "Dr. W. H. Alexander's Healing Oil: For dandruff, scalp troubles, burns, cuts, sprains, sore throat and chest colds (rub externally), eczema, tetter, sore feet, corns, mange on dogs, harness galls, all flesh wounds."

Here began my ideas of illness and healing.

'JESUS LOVES
THE LITTLE CHILDREN'

In the Sunday School of the First Baptist Church, we sang:

Jesus loves the little children,
All the children of the world,
Red and yellow, black and white,
They are precious in His sight.
Jesus loves the little children of the world.

At Christmas time, on a Sunday afternoon, we white children in the primary grades sat on one side of the room with a present in each of our laps. Many of our mothers were there, stirring about before joining us. A fully decorated Christmas tree stood at one end of the large room. In front of it was a table with punch and cookies.

The door to the room opened, and a line of black children our age entered with several of their mothers. How the group traveled to the First Baptist Church I never knew, for few cars were evident in Goose Hollow or the other black neighborhoods in our community.

The black children—boys in starched white shirts and girls in stiffly ironed dresses—sat with their mothers in perfect silence along the opposite wall. No one spoke on our side of the room either.

The white teacher moved to a podium next to the punch table to welcome everybody. She read a few verses from the Bible's nativity story. One at a time the name of each white child was called. The script called for each of us to proceed to a spot before the table of refreshments. The name of a black child was then called to come forward and receive a present from us. Each white child said, "Merry Christmas." Each black child replied, "Thank you," and we returned to our seats.

Our mothers shopped for the presents. Mine never showed me what she bought, and since the presents were not opened at our gathering, I never knew the contents of the boxes. I suspect most of it was clothing, since there were no telltale rattles when boxes were shaken.

After the exchange of presents our teacher led us in singing "Silent Night" as she accompanied on the piano. White mothers passed out cookies and cups of punch to the children of each race, each group staying on its side of an imaginary line bisecting that room. The black children maintained a mannerly silence, while we white children chatted among ourselves. After the black children were ushered out, a noisier conversation among the white children prevailed until we sang more Christmas carols and then went home.

A rosy glow abounded at home as we "haves" shared whatever largesse was wrapped and packaged by our parents. When we presented the gifts at Sunday School it was charity indeed, but with a clear implication that giver and receiver were not to mingle. And the recipient of that charity was to remain docile and remember his or her place quietly at the far reach of that malignant pecking order.

When I was 12 or thereabouts, *The LaGrange Daily News* carried a brief item about a hit-and-run accident in which a car carrying three white men through a black neighborhood had struck a child. The car had stopped, and one of its occupants had run back to check on the victim. "It's only a nigger," he was quoted as yelling back to the driver of the car. The three sped off. I never saw a follow-up story.

Thirty years later, in another city, as I took a medical history from a black foundry worker with hypertension and emphysema, I learned that LaGrange, Georgia, was the place of his birth and upbringing. I spoke of our shared birthplace. He smiled and nodded. As the years passed and he and I built that social structure known as rapport, I asked him what he recalled of that time and that place.

He had lived on the other side of town on East Depot Street. His mother had worked as cook and maid for a white family, and his father tended white people's yards.

"I don't think much about it. I know we had enough to eat," he said. He recalled often going with his father on weekends to do pick-up work around the yards that his father mowed and raked. Sometimes he did inside cleaning. He remembered eating especially well on those days when his father's employer passed plates of food to them, which they were to eat on the back steps.

As he grew into junior high years his mother warned him repeatedly to avoid white people; it was best not to look them in the face.

"Did you have lights and running water?" I asked.

"I think we had water, but we used kerosene lamps," he said.

He was allowed to go downtown only with his father or mother. Each Sunday his family went to church, which he recalled lasting two or three hours.

He was drafted in World War II, serving as a cook in Europe. After the war he was hesitant to return to LaGrange; besides, there was talk of better jobs in the factories and foundries of Chattanooga. Slowly, he progressed from janitorial work to casting. He spoke with pride of the house that he and his nurse's aide wife had purchased.

Cigarettes and the acrid fumes of the foundry progressively attacked his lungs. He worked on, despite shortness of breath, finally earning his pension at age 65. By that time he could only walk short distances quite slowly.

My patient and I shared a place of birth and a hometown, but we could just as well have grown up on separate planets.

"Didn't you ever get angry?" I asked him during one of his visits to my office.

"I never thought much about it," he said. "It would not have done any good."

He worked hard, and I never saw him angry or cynical. He developed carcinoma of the lung and, with the quiet courage that had driven his life, approached a death which occurred a few weeks following diagnosis.

Although town fathers disallowed public violence against black residents of LaGrange, they were treated as if they were never entirely within focus. Conversation between whites was directed as if a witnessing black citizen were simply not present and, in any event, incapable of comprehending what was spoken. A simpler, almost childlike speech was directed at black men and women. To questions about wretched housing and schools, the standard replies given to children were that the black people paid no taxes or drank up all their money. Hence, they deserved poor living conditions.

One black woman had special status in those long-ago days. Her name was Charlie, and she may have been my first real friend. Certainly I loved her. She was a licensed practical nurse and the person to be called whenever a seriously ill member of LaGrange's gentry was to be nursed back to health. Judges, physicians, storekeepers, their children, and their wives looked to her for a special kind of intensive care as they convalesced in hospital or home from major illness or surgery.

Her speech was precisely articulated, pitched in a rich alto. She never seemed to age. Her handwriting could have served as a model for any primary classroom. She knew American history and closely followed current events.

Often, she was my baby sitter, a strong and loving presence. She read to me and told me of the evil of the Nazis as World War II broke out. She alerted me to the atrocities committed by Americans as well. She told me that white people and black people were loved equally by God, and I believed her.

I saw her at various bedsides, and she used her nursing skills well into her 70s. Was it her voice that conveyed power and gentleness or some special healing sense that she brought to the sickroom? The notion she always transmitted was that the situation was under control and there was nothing to fear. Once I was present as she encouraged one of my aunts, weakened by recent surgery, to move from bed to chair. Coaxing and encouraging and ever so gently lifting, she guided her patient into the cushioned seat. She fluffed the pillow behind her head. She combed her hair. She guided a cup of warm tea to her patient's lips, encouraging and congratulating her continuously. This was the voice and presence of an angel.

One day in 1980 my family and I visited her. Now retired, she lived in a modest white home in the black neighborhood of her youth. By then I was married and father of four sons. I had been in medical practice for more than ten years.

"Cliffie," she said, "I want you to have these." She gave each of our sons a silver dollar and a bag of pecans to my wife and me. She had picked the nuts from trees in her yard and shelled them. We sat in her living room and drank Coca-Colas and spoke of earlier times. She told me which citizens I knew in my youth had died and who was recently sick and how the town's medical center had progressed. Framed pictures of Martin Luther King Jr. and John F. Kennedy sat atop her television set. She lived into her 90s.

Did she harbor deep hostility or sorrow? I never asked her, but I sensed not. Even today, when I hear the term "angel," it is her image that immediately comes to mind. To the bedside of the sick she brought a serene power. To her community, not yet freed of the spiritual bonds of slavery and racial injustice, she spoke, in her way, of all our shared vulnerabilities and aspirations. To me, she brought first knowledge of what the terms "brotherhood" and "sisterhood" meant when applied beyond my biological family.

A BOY'S LEG

The small black boy, maybe five or six years old, stood sobbing on his front porch. His wire-thin extremities spoke of a life of inadequate nutrition. A charred left leg extended from his dirtied short pants.

Many of LaGrange's black citizens lived in pocket ghettos—small enclaves interspersed among the white neighborhoods—where the men worked to keep yards and the women cooked, ironed, and cleaned for their white employers. The 30 or so unpainted frame shacks of Goose Hollow formed one such enclave. These houses had neither electric power nor indoor plumbing; some shared outhouses. An eroded red clay street wound through this community.

Our threesome of white eight-year-olds had taken a shortcut through the hollow following a pick-up baseball game late on a Sunday afternoon. Time for our suppers was at hand. Our curiosity forced a pause as we saw the boy. I asked the lady who appeared behind the tattered screen of the door what had happened to cause this injury. She replied that the boy had fallen in a fire days earlier. I asked if she had taken the boy to a hospital or doctor. She shook her head, "No."

A closer look showed thin rivulets of pus separating the charred flakes of skin on the boy's leg. A yellow salve had been applied. We drew back, speechless, from this sight. Our route out of the hollow led us through the backyard of an elderly white physician. I knocked on the side door of his house; his wife opened the door part way. I asked to see the doctor. She firmly explained that he was sleeping, and he was not to be disturbed. I explained to her what we three had seen and that the injured boy needed help. She retorted that people in the hollow had no money and never paid their bills. I was instructed to direct the mother to take her child to the hospital. I ran back to Goose Hollow to relay the message.

Two weeks later my late afternoon play concluded, and I retraced my earlier shortcut through Goose Hollow. No one was on the boy's porch. The house appeared closed. I asked a neighbor about the boy. I was told that he had died. Anger and grief are my adult responses to that grim news in that forsaken place. I do not recall my response as a little boy, except that I carry forever a memory of sadness and learned for the first time what injustice was all about.

CLARA

She was large-boned, obese, and ebony-skinned, and she appeared perpetually tired. She lived on Callaway Line, a two-block-long unpaved black neighborhood which linked white-only Gordon Street and South Lewis Street. She was probably 35 but walked slowly up a gently inclined driveway to our duplex like a much older woman. Her facial expression was emotionally neutral. She had huge breasts unfettered by a bra until my mother convinced her that her back might hurt less if she wore such an undergarment.

Clara said little, except to reply "Y's'm" and "No'm" in response to questions. Her ten-year-old son lived with her in a shack with a tarpapered roof. Her husband had left her and was reported to live in Detroit. The houses on her street allegedly were owned by a physician. Only a few men were ever in evidence along this street. The eldest women remained home and could be seen washing clothes in large iron pots over open fires at road's edge. One especially large woman served as the head of this neighborhood.

At night the neighborhood was remarkable for its quietness. Cracks of pale yellow kerosene-generated light might outline a single window. Sometimes, late on a Saturday night, a police siren would pierce the quiet. My uncle, who was a policeman, spoke of occasional fights in the ghetto that ended in stabbings. When the police arrived, they negotiated with the large female neighborhood director to determine what had happened and who might be responsible. The combatants would be nowhere in sight. This impoverished colony within our community had its own laws and codes of behavior.

Clara received seven dollars and fifty cents for each week's work at our house. She ironed, cleaned, mopped, and washed our clothes. Sometimes, she prepared a meal. She ate leftovers in our kitchen or in our backyard. My mother gave her hand-me-downs for herself and her son. She departed for home late each afternoon, except Sundays, when her work was finished by late morning. One Sunday morning Clara was late for work. There was a faint knock on our front door. Clara's son stood there. "Mamma won't be at work today. She's been shot."

From the police, my parents learned the following: Clara had gone with her date to a club the night before. After too many drinks she and her male friend returned to her cabin. Police were summoned by neighbors after gunshots were heard. Clara was taken away by ambulance and her companion was arrested. He was described as too inebriated to escape. I was told that Clara had been shot in the liver. Her condition was poor. She barely clung to life. The nurse on Clara's ward did not permit my mother to visit.

Two days later her white doctor sent word to my parents through his child that he could not be expected to treat Clara any further unless he was paid. Later that same day Clara died in the hospital.

My mother took my sister and me to part of Clara's funeral, which was held in a tiny bare-walled chapel across town in another black neighborhood. Her closed wooden casket rested in front of the pulpit, from which a minister spoke loudly. A hymn was sung and Scripture was read. I recall women standing and wailing as their arms moved slowly above their heads. After an hour or so we left quietly as the congregation stood to sing again.

Another family on Callaway Line took in Clara's son. Clara's husband returned to LaGrange for her funeral. In his neatly tailored suit and Panama hat he contrasted sharply with the overalls and faded funeral attire of the other mourners. He departed a week later with a young woman in tow. Clara's assailant received a one-year sentence for involuntary manslaughter. Within days of the burial, Clara's cabin had been rented to another family.

That blighted neighborhood disappeared years ago. The street is paved and renamed, and there is no visible evidence of the people who once lived there. I doubt that a former resident would have any interest in seeking out the place where he once lived. Far in the future an archaeologist, digging beneath the concrete of driveways and finished basements, might find evidence of septic tanks or ashes from remote fires or even part of a glass chimney attached to a kerosene lantern. He could only guess at the sorrow fading even now in the archaeology of memory.

A LARGE PRESENCE

On the frontispiece of Uncle Rube's 1885 *Science and Art of Midwifery* were these penciled notes.

Treatment of eclampsia (Jones) 1895:

1. When called to patient with symptoms of Ec., either bleed one to two pints and purge and give hot bath to get rid of poison or deliver by force.

2. When eclampsia is present and labor has not commenced: dilate the os, which takes from one to two hours and deliver the child, or else bleed and if patient condition is good may let pregnancy go on. Give KCl during convulsion or during operation.

3. When labor commenced: hasten delivery. Purge and sweat as necessary. Chloral Morphine no good as simply adds more poison to the blood. Get rid of poison.

Inside this volume, which came to me after my great uncle's death, was a page from a pocket ledger, listing charges of a dollar to a dollar and a half for clinic visits. Serving as a marker between other pages was a receipt for strychnine.

Reuben O'Neal, a general practitioner in a west Georgia cotton mill town, practiced until his late 90s. Certainly he was 90 when I last visited him at his office.

It was late afternoon and his final patient of the day, a thin, wraith-like lady, shuffled slowly out the waiting room door. He lowered his huge frame into a waiting room chair and began asking questions. How was I doing in my newly established practice? What kind of patients and problems did I encounter? What textbooks did I find most useful? Then he sought my opinion on a new drug or two.

His aged nurse said her goodbyes as she moved slowly to the door, locking it behind her.

"I mainly see old folks now. They like to visit and talk," he said.

Most of his patients had died; the remainder had grown older with him. He ticked off the names of several mutual acquaintances who had recently passed away. He was quick to refer to younger physicians anyone with an ailment that might require more intensive therapy than he could provide in his office. He no longer visited the hospital.

He had been obese from my earliest memory. For years, I had noted a rounded, firm-appearing protuberant lesion on one side of his neck. A tumor? A bony structure? He had to be aware of the presence of this mass. Had the growth been important, surely it would have killed him by now.

As the light yellowed and was divided into bars by the slats of the Venetian blinds, we traded family news: his granddaughters and great-grandchildren, my parents and children. We spoke of illness and tragedy that had befallen people whose names I could no longer link to faces.

Uncle Rube finished medical school just in time to join the American Expeditionary Force to France in World War I. He brought home an ornate ceremonial German helmet with a brass spike at its crown. Despite my repeated questions during my boyhood he volunteered little information about his wartime experiences. He told me once about lengthy surgeries of the wounded under difficult conditions. Another time he spoke of the influenza epidemic at war's end, which claimed more casualties than the battlefield. When I asked about the cause of paralysis in an elderly man who was driven about town by his wife, Uncle Rube explained that the man had been a victim of a poison gas attack in the first Great War.

Back in LaGrange, Uncle Rube did it all: delivering hundreds of babies, treating major and minor illnesses and injuries, and performing lots of general surgery. My family lived in a duplex near his home. Repeatedly at night I saw his car—a wonderful 1940 DeSoto with steel "eyelids" which raised when the headlights were turned on—as he drove hurriedly to the hospital. This was my first introduction to the mystique of medicine. On one night's ride he ran over my dog, Spot, who had the dangerous habit of sleeping on the warmer pavement of the street.

Uncle Rube defined presence for me. At those times when I saw him at the bedside of sick relatives, his deep voice was slow and measured, his attention focused and intense. After taking a pulse he continued to hold the patient's hand while asking questions or delivering advice. In that era, physicians carried black bags. This was a sign of both mystery and authority, conferring professional rank in the same way a nurse's cap designated members of that profession. A stethoscope, a folding mercury manometer, a small case of surgical probes and forceps, suturing material, bottles, and syringes—these were the neatly arrayed contents of the magical and scuffed black leather bag.

Medical offices of that day were starkly white. All physicians' offices shared the same pungent, antiseptic aroma, almost formalin-like in its nasal sting. Blindfolded, any child or adult would know immediately upon entry that he was in a doctor's office.

Beyond the stark waiting room of Uncle Rube's office, all was shiny and white: white tile, white walls, and white glass-doored cabinets. His nurse and receptionist were white-clad as well, and he wore a heavily starched white coat. Each morning as he left home his wife pinned a fresh flower to the lapel of his suit coat, which he wore whenever he stepped from his office.

When I was ten I stepped on a nail, which penetrated the sole of my canvas shoe and drove deep into my foot. Because I remembered a cousin who fought osteomyelitis for years after a similar injury and almost lost his foot, I assumed the worst. No one was home that afternoon, so I limped to Uncle Rube's office alone, fearing that by day's end I would lose my leg. I maintained my bravery as I explained to his receptionist what had happened, even while his nurse removed my shoe and sock in the examining room. But this brave front was to dissolve as this large, great uncle eased into the room and examined my foot. I do not remember the words, except for their softness and comfort. I do recall two injections but, because he gave them himself, they did not hurt badly. I was instructed how to soak my foot in hot water with Epsom salts and to stop by the office two days later for a re-check. Uncle Rube's authority ensured my recovery. I worried about my foot no longer.

My first job—I was, perhaps, eight—was in his employ. On Saturday mornings his wife, Aunt Lelia, cranked up her LaSalle sedan to take me on collection rounds through the villages that surrounded each cotton mill. I earned a dollar each Saturday.

Each cotton mill, at least in that part of the country, formed the nucleus of its own community. Large, drab, brick structures operated constantly. Whistles heard widely throughout the town signaled the beginnings and endings of eight-hour shifts as well as meal times. Identical, small frame dwellings lined surrounding streets. Often, both husband and wife in each house worked in the mills, alternating their shifts if young children were at home.

The houses where I collected shared a common floor plan. An equal number of wooden steps led to a covered porch, roomy enough to accommodate a cane-bottomed rocking chair or two. A knock on the door and my spiel would begin: "Collect for Dr. O'Neal." From the doorway I had glimpses into dozens of homes. Many were neat; some were in total disarray. I was greeted by women in kerchiefs and terry cloth robes and sack-like work dresses. I saw children, washed and dirty, playing inside in winter, playing in the small front yards in summer. Occasionally, I recognized a classmate. Sometimes, I saw startling poverty in houses with multiple children.

Payment might be fifty cents or one dollar always placed in an envelope. Sometimes payment might be two, four, or six eggs, and once I was given a freshly plucked chicken.

After thanking the debtor I delivered the payment to Aunt Lelia for entry in a large ledger before proceeding to the next house.

Uncle Rube served at least two terms as mayor of that community. Sometimes when I stopped at his home, Aunt Lelia would tell me of his exhaustion from the previous night's work, and she would warn me to be quiet because, for now, he was sleeping. I could visit him later. If work was quiet on a summer evening, he might take me to watch the Troupers play baseball in the Class D Georgia-Alabama League.

Legends abounded, the makings of some I even witnessed. My favorite concerned the bootlegger who, finally convicted, beseeched Uncle Rube to provide care for the whiskey-maker's wife and children during the time when he would be away in prison. Uncle Rube provided this care for two years. Following the release of the distiller from prison, a case of whiskey—the bonded variety—arrived at my great uncle's home every Christmas Day for years, courtesy of the grateful husband-father.

Only once did I make hospital rounds with him. I was in medical school. By then, Uncle Rube had stopped performing surgery. There were a half dozen patients, one with a stroke, another with pneumonia, another recovering from heart failure. All were as old as he. The deep, slowly paced voice was the same I had heard at the time of my foot injury. After each examination we sat for a few minutes to visit before we moved on. Did I detect a hint of pride when he introduced me each time?

On the day of his funeral there was insufficient time to drive from Chattanooga to LaGrange. I stopped instead in Atlanta to visit my Aunt Ida, a widow in her 80s, whose frail health prevented her traveling to the service. As Uncle Rube had been patriarch of his generation, so she—his niece—was matriarch of hers. They had been especially close as he, the professional, and she, the nurturer, had tended to the needs of sick relatives spread over three generations. Whenever a close relative was sick, my aunt rode the Greyhound bus to LaGrange each weekend to spend two days assisting in the care of the patient.

My usually calm aunt was agitated and, for the first time ever in my presence, tearful.

She asked, "What will we do, what will we do?" We sat in a living room surrounded by her African violets, antimacassars, and dozens of pictures of four generations of Cleavelands and O'Neals. We talked and sipped coffee. I held her hand and reassured her that we would be well.

CALOMEL DAYS

People in my hometown had a fixation on regular bowel function. Conversation among adults often included a guarded query or recommendation regarding the latest laxative or cathartic. Perhaps the meat and potato-oriented diet of that day contained too little of the fiber which we now revere. In any event a predictable, daily bowel movement was regarded as a prerequisite for a good life. "Ex-Lax," "Sal Hepatica," ("Ipana for the smile of beauty, Sal Hepatica for the smile of health," the radio commercial intoned), and a brown tablet called "Caroid and Bile Salts" were best sellers among the many over-the-counter preparations for recalcitrant bowels. One or more of these preparations could be found beside the kitchen sink or inside the medicine cabinet of most homes. If a child acted grumpy or the least out of sorts, he could expect a dose of milk of magnesia. If no improvement were forthcoming, a teaspoon or two of dreaded castor oil was the final mood and bowel modifier. Fear of the ultimate treatment caused many children of that day and place to feign vigorous health and a smiling disposition even if they felt quite the contrary.

Each spring, as the azaleas and mimosas bloomed, the dreaded calomel dose was administered. The popular view held that various poisons accumulated in the gut throughout the fall and winter. These had to be expelled before one could fully enter into the activities of the new season. A tablet of calomel, mercurous chloride, was the purgative of choice. Typically, a Saturday in early spring was picked. One tablet for children, two for adults were administered. After three to four hours of increasing borborygmi and bloating, the fecal explosions would begin. Family members competed for use of the toilet in the single-bathroom households.

The Random House Dictionary of the English Language traces the word *calomel* from *calomelas,* which is derived in turn from the Greek *kalos* (fair) plus *melas* (black), because manufacture of the substance involved a chemical conversion from a white substance to a black substance. Actually, I believe the ancient Greeks simply knew what human administration of the drug would do to the recipient's humor.

Sunday dawned. Children and adults, all somewhat pale and subdued, proceeded to Sunday School and church. Following Sunday dinner the rigors of the preceding day were relegated to the winter's history and life moved on.

DURHAM

1954

PREMEDICAL study at Duke University meant a major in either chemistry or zoology. A premedical advisor in my freshman years emphasized that heavy-duty science should form the core of my scholarly activity. I would need a grade point average of 3.5 or better to qualify for medical school. Occasional meetings of a premedical club re-emphasized the importance of high grades in science courses. Thus began a systematized grind.

In a demanding curriculum, two courses—comparative anatomy and organic chemistry—had the reputation of being the steepest hurdles. In the semester-long course of comparative anatomy, we meticulously dissected our way up the phylogenetic tree, learning along the way far too much about the anatomy of sharks and cats. Impossible schedules in the laboratory required nights and Saturdays to complete projects. Organic chemistry, spread over two semesters, maintained the same pace with little time for us to determine whether we actually enjoyed the subject or not. A "C plus" in my first semester briefly forced me to think of other career choices; I knew none. A "B plus" in the following semester saved the day. The two courses served a role comparable to basic training in the military, and the instructors exhibited many of the attributes of drill sergeants: pushing, upbraiding, shaping, challenging. No course in medical school was to be as demanding.

I doubt that a student majoring in liberal arts would have gained entry to medical school in that day. The university required a scattering of liberal arts courses for science majors. Sustained inquiry into the humanities was not feasible. If chemistry seemed most of the time a monotonous chore, my brief forays into literature and history were sheer delights. Much of the required premedical curriculum seemed to be a necessary evil, a string of demanding, mechanistic courses required to enter the monastery of medicine.

Now I realize the incompleteness of medical education based solely upon science. Medicine is not simply a branch of chemistry or the biological sciences. Clinicians especially live among stories: those of their patients and their colleagues and those that seek expression within their own souls. Imaginative literature has taught me more about my patients than any course or text in science. Patients are not diseases but human beings with complex histories who happen to have experienced illness or injury. It is literature that permits us to feel our way into our patients' experiences. Without this awareness, we are at risk of processing rather than treating those who seek our help.

My long-standing acne reflected the tides of stress, flaring at times of examination or before a big social weekend. A nurse at Student Health referred me to the dermatology section of the Duke Clinic during one such exacerbation. Oftentimes, undergraduate students were treated perfunctorily. The dermatology professor, whom I visited repeatedly during the next three years, was different, a smiling and rotund man who engaged me in honest conversation as he used radiation, various creams and drying agents, and occasionally metallic probes in my fight against imagined or real disfigurement. He extolled the benefits of his clinical specialty, emphasizing the lack of night and weekend call and the gratitude of his patients.

Once, in my sophomore year, a searing anal pain prompted another visit to the Student Health office. The examining resident told me I had a thrombosed external hemorrhoid and arranged an appointment in a surgical clinic for that afternoon. At the appointed place and hour, I was issued a surgical gown. This garment has not evolved since medicine's earliest days. Doubtless, Hippocrates had something to do with the design of the foreshortened garment, which in its devious design places the patient immediately on the defensive. Thus gowned, I was led into a room marked "Minor Procedures." The nurse directed me to lie over a large wedge with my bare bottom exposed and aimed at the door. A surgical resident who never introduced himself entered, mumbled a few words, and prepared to incise the painful protuberance. Just then, the door opened behind me. I glanced around to see an instructor with three nursing students—one of whom I had recently dated—enter the room to observe. Just then, the scalpel struck the nonanesthetized tissue. Oh, pain! Oh, wretched flare of acne!

I returned to Duke Hospital on a Saturday in 1963 to interview for an internship on the medical service. I was scheduled to meet a professor at his office in early afternoon. I parked my aging, finned Plymouth at the far end of a parking lot and apprehensively began to walk to the hospital. I heard a scuffle just ahead and, as I rounded a pickup truck, came upon a man sitting astride a young girl whom he was beating in the face. A woman, perhaps the girl's mother, stood motionless a few feet away, her face covered by her hands. The assailant whirled toward me, as surprised as I was. He bolted. The child ran to the woman, who picked her up and fled in the opposite direction. I ran to the hospital in search of a policeman. Just outside the hospital entrance, I was spun around by a hand on my shoulder. It was the man.

"If you say anything or report this, I'll kill you," he said.

I dodged away and, inside the hospital lobby, I called the campus police. Within minutes, an officer came, and then another, to record my report.

I explained my tardiness to a sympathetic interviewer. Our chat went well, despite my pounding tachycardia. As I left Duke Hospital an hour later I recognized one of the policemen. He told me that the child beater had been apprehended. He had been discharged from the psychiatric ward of the Durham VA Hospital only that morning. The little girl was his daughter and was being treated in the emergency room.

Sheer chance brought the little girl and me together. Sheer chance possibly spared her serious physical injury or even death, at least for a time. This would not be the last time I would witness a chance act with far-reaching consequences.

OXFORD

1958-1961

W E students stood as the college Fellows arrived at high table. After the Lord's Prayer in Latin we began our predictable dinner of Brussels sprouts or cabbage, boiled potatoes, and some form of beef or mutton. The diners at high table, which was situated on a dais, were served from ancient silver plates by a butler who kept their wine goblets filled throughout the repast. The 180 Scholars and Commoners sat on benches at three long parallel tables. We drank beer with our meals. I was nervous, for my first tutorial would follow this meal.

Still wearing the short, black academic gown of a Commoner, I knocked at the door of my tutor's quarters situated off the main quadrangle of my college. In a brief meeting one week earlier he had assigned, with little explanation, the topic of transmission of impulses along the nerve fibers of the giant squid. He mentioned two references that I might find helpful. These led to dozens of other papers and textbooks. Quickly, the topic was out of hand. I felt out of my league and believed that it was not possible to compress this large body of knowledge into the typed pages of a single essay. In the best tradition of procrastination, I completed my essay just prior to dinner.

Ushering me into a too warm room, Bob Torrance—I did not dare use his first name until after my graduation—was a large and imposing presence. I was frankly intimidated by his size and the breadth of his knowledge of physiology. As my three years progressed, I came to regard him as a gentle giant who used his scientific expertise almost apologetically, asking, "Oh, really?" if my point was wrong or stating "Nicely done" if an essay were especially pertinent.

He directed me to an upholstered chair placed before an open fireplace and offered me a glass of port, which I accepted. The small sitting room was bounded by bookshelves on every wall. Battling somnolence, I launched into my paper. Following an hour of recitation and discussion, my physician-tutor, before dismissing me, encouraged me to attend a concert rendition of *The Magic Flute* the following Sunday afternoon.

This was preclinical study at England's Oxford University. A scholarship had directed me there, changing my plans to enter an American medical school after graduation from Duke.

Oxford's medical curriculum began with two years of physiology, anatomy, and biochemistry. An additional one to two years of work toward a degree in physiology or biochemistry preceded a half year of pathology, microbiology, and pharmacology. Three and a half years of clinical study followed. Students from England began this course of study immediately after completing the equivalent of American high school.

Eight-week terms featured tutorial, lab, and lecture. Tutorials were intense and focused, and those of each term covered, in a systematic fashion, the principles of an area such as pulmonary physiology or carbohydrate metabolism. We might be assigned to a tutor outside our college to benefit from that teacher's expertise in a particular branch of physiology or biochemistry. Laboratories resembled their American counterparts, though they were much more modestly equipped. Anatomy labs were quite different in that we were free to dissect whenever it was most convenient for our team. Lab assistants, often surgeons completing their professional qualifications, were always present to advise and to explain why no team's cadaver ever resembled the pictures and descriptions of the dissecting manuals. Our first hospital rounds correlated our dissections with patients whose diseases or injuries afflicted the body part we were currently studying. Our work was demanding but never harried.

Terms were separated by 6-week-long vacations at Christmas and Easter, and a 16-week summer hiatus. Prior to each we visited the tutors who were to supervise the following term's work to obtain our reading lists. These books and articles would serve as the foundation for the next segments in anatomy, physiology, and biochemistry. It was presumed that we would read all of the material before our return.

While British students returned to their homes in London, Yorkshire, and Glasgow, we North Americans hit the road, sometimes as visitors to Cornish homes or Welsh farms, sometimes hitchhiking to warmer parts of the continent, our bags of books in tow. Before each departure we appeared before the Senior Fellows of our college. My academic tutor would comment on my progress, or lack thereof, and enumerate his expectations for the coming term. The college also assigned each student a "moral tutor," who would report if we had run afoul of any rule or custom.

Each college comprised its own separate academic island within the university. Students from all disciplines— law, medicine, classics, history, philosophy—lived and dined in the college. Tutors for each discipline were the college's Fellows who, if bachelors, usually occupied apartments within the college. At dinner in the hall, with its high vaulted ceiling, we would be "sconced" if we were overheard talking shop. A student so challenged could either buy a round of beer for everyone at his long table or down three pints of beer from a large silver flagon without removing the vessel from his lips. If the latter feat were accomplished, the challenger had to pay for the beer.

Each college fielded a full array of athletic teams. Should a team fill up in one sport, another team would simply be created. We medical students rowed in eights, played tennis, or took up such new sports as field hockey and rugby. I learned that I did not have to be a semi-professional to play college sports. I also learned that one could play any sport in any weather; the English postpone nothing for fog, rain, or cold.

Music, drama, endless bridge games, and searches for the perfect pub occupied hours each week. A friend attending U.S. medical school described in his letters to me a radically different way of life:

one of perpetual work. Neither he nor his classmates ever seemed happy. By contrast I could count on several afternoons or evenings each week for nonmedical activities. It was indeed possible to be both medical student and human being.

Our rooms in college were organized around staircases that did not connect to each other. My first-floor pair of rooms sat in the corner of the New Buildings (circa 1881) in St. John Baptist College (founded 1555). My room had a single electric heating coil and its function depended on a steady diet of shillings fed into its meter. An electric blanket brought from home preserved my warmth at night in a perpetually cold and damp building.

A manservant, or "scout," looked after the rooms and students on each staircase. My scout was a former POW who had been captured at Dunkirk. Thoroughly versed in the intricate customs of Oxford, the university, Fred also knew everything about Oxford, the city. He pointed with pride to a picture of the University servants' soccer team on which he had played prior to Army service. Anything I needed, he knew where I might buy it at a reduced price. When in my third year I returned to Oxford with my new wife, he extended to us the same knowledge and generous hospitality. After I left St. John's we exchanged Christmas cards. A few years later tuberculosis, which he had acquired while a prisoner of the Germans, flared, and he lost a year of work. When I next saw him 17 years after completing my Oxford studies, he recognized me at once. As we drank a cup of tea, he showed me the small notebook in which he had listed every student he had ever served, with notes of their later activities. He died at home of a ruptured aortic aneurysm in the mid-1980s.

A single bathroom, accessible only after a walk or run across the open square, served the residents of my college's quadrangle. This encouraged increased nocturnal bladder control, especially in cold weather. The quad's single bathtub required a reservation.

On spring days St. John's extensive gardens exploded into bloom, and carpets of grass defined the superlative of green. We took our books outside half reading, half dreaming. A relaxed float on the Thames or a stroll through the meadows of Christ Church or Magdalen Colleges would immediately restore a sinking spirit. These were glorious days.

Our first two years of work culminated in a formal examination, part I of the bachelor of medicine. Written, lab, and oral testing provided a measure of our efforts to that point. Our third year was devoted to physiology, especially that of the nervous system. The format remained the same. We worked hard and played with equal devotion. A four-day-long examination closed this happy chapter.

I returned to the United States to complete medical studies at Johns Hopkins. The two experiences were worlds apart. Both approaches to medical education seemed to produce equally competent physicians in the end.

A friend defined her Anglican religion as "Christianity-light: demanding but with just a little less guilt." By analogy, Oxford was "medical school-light: demanding with just a little less guilt."

THE CARE OF STRANGERS

I was a stranger in a strange country, and I was quite ill. Prior to setting foot in England I joined future classmates in a trip to the Brussels World's Fair of 1958. In one of the venues of that spectacle I acquired a Salmonella time bomb, which was to go off three days later when I reached London.

Initially, I had diarrhea, which I attacked with bottles of Kaopectate. I ran through the panoply of home remedies of my upbringing: clear liquids, toast, pinches of table salt. A pharmacist, or "chemist" as they are called in England, concocted a bitter liquid tasting of paregoric, which he promised would stem the tide.

But I became progressively sicker. I experienced dizziness whenever I stood. Fevers and sweats interrupted my sleep. One night I had recurrent hallucinations. I now passed blood and mucus. For the first time in my life, I felt that I was dying. I was too weak to get out of bed. The proprietor of the tiny hotel knocked. The cleaning lady, whom I had not seen, had informed him that I seemed very ill. After confirming this he called his physician who came at the noon hour to check me. I needed hospitalization. He called an ambulance, and I was off to the Western Fever Hospital.

The West Indian physician who met the ambulance commented

upon my peculiar accent. Though we spoke the same words in the same syntax, our dialects rendered us almost incommunicative. Blood was taken and I was hooked to intravenous fluids and admitted to an isolation room.

Each morning the nurse awakened the entire ward at 4:30 by turning on bright lights. An aide brought me a pan of hot water, soap, a towel, and a cup of tea. Breakfast arrived at 6:00 A.M. A professor and his retinue saw me each mid-morning. They contemplated the clinical chart but never examined me. At supper on that first day a glass of dark, frothy liquid at room temperature accompanied my meal. This was Guinness stout, preferred only by the heartiest imbibers in the pubs in the United Kingdom. Someone had decided stout would do me good. The first swallow reminded me of a bitter American patent medicine called Creomulsion. I dutifully drank the rest and remembered nothing until the next day. I never acquired a taste for the ale, despite a nightly serving.

I was not allowed magazines or newspapers. My only entertainment was a small primitive radio, which received a single band of the BBC. A glass wall separated me from other beds in which lay patients with polio. All lights were turned off in the early evening.

On the third day my IV fluids were stopped. I could eat without cramps and nausea. The Oxford director of my scholarship program phoned the hospital and inquired of my needs. Through the nurse I relayed my desire for something—anything—to read. He visited the following day bearing a gift of *The Brothers Karamazov*.

Several days later, pale and thinner than usual, I was discharged from the hospital. The house doctor told me that I had been infected with *Salmonella sonnei* and that I would be weak for a while but would soon be okay. I was.

"Socialized medicine," it was called in America. Even in our present-day debates regarding health care, the British National Health Service is presented as something evil and insensitive to the needs of the sick. Granted, the system has been progressively weakened over the years by a pattern of inadequate funding and cumbersome administration, but the NHS does ensure every citizen of the United Kingdom predictable, accessible, and essential health services. My later contacts with NHS physicians for treatment of lesser ailments at Oxford reaffirmed the clinical skills intrinsic to the program.

I witnessed this system again in 1990 when I spent the day with a British friend and classmate, now a gastroenterologist, in his endoscopy suite in an NHS Hospital. The staff was expert, the equipment more sophisticated than any I had seen in my own American hospital. At mid-morning a rain storm arrived and in a few minutes multiple drops of water dripped into our room. Quickly, the nurse covered the equipment with plastic, commenting that this happened whenever it rained. My friend explained that repeated entreaties to repair the roof were ignored. Clearly, the NHS needed sustained major infusions of capital.

In 1958 I, a student visitor with no insurance card—and none was ever demanded—was treated expertly and kindly in a hospital, at no cost to me, by doctors and nurses who taught me more than any of us had reckoned.

BALTIMORE

1961-1964

AMERICAN cities show an amazing capacity for reinventing themselves, at least superficially. Baltimore's harbor front, with its promenades, aquarium, upscale shops, and Camden Yards baseball stadium, now regularly attracts relaxed crowds of citizens and visitors alike. The contrast with the same area in the early 1960s is quite stark. Faded buildings, unswept and potholed streets, and sullen faces greeted the visitor, who was best advised to avoid the area altogether after dark. There and in East Baltimore aggressive female prostitutes harassed even the most innocent of passersby. Elsewhere in the city communities of Germans, Czechs, African Americans, Poles, and Chinese created a patchwork of accent and custom. At the perimeter stood giant steel plants belching forth smoke and fumes, while a few miles away mansions on manicured lawns evoked images of old, unreconstructed Southern graciousness.

Just north of the harbor the historic dome of the Johns Hopkins Hospital protruded from a skyline not yet tall enough to obscure it. This medical island sat in the middle of an impoverished, largely black neighborhood where violence lurked always just beneath the surface. On the sidewalks dripped trails of dried blood pointed to the emergency room. Students and housestaff either lived within the compound or rented apartments in partially reclaimed tenements at inflated prices. The hospital attracted, by convenience, destitute neighbors when they were sick or injured and, by reputation, the well-insured and rich from home and abroad. A tall statue of Jesus reached out tentatively at one entrance to all who entered.

Johnny Unitas had led the Baltimore Colts to the NFL Championship, giving the city a sense of increased worth among its peers. The Baltimore Orioles had finally learned how to win as Brooks Robinson began a remarkable career at third base. Sports finally gave the city reasons for pride, which transcended economic and ethnic barriers. Spiro Agnew, as he campaigned for the top elective office in Baltimore County, lambasted the established political machine and promised fresh leadership and honest government. He met both goals, at least in Maryland.

For medical students, and even more so for housestaff, Hopkins was comparable to a large cave from which only occasional participation with and glimpses of the larger community could be experienced. The institution's ethic was based on unremitting work; the satisfaction of ever fully completing a task was seldom enjoyed. It was a workaholic's idea of heaven. On clinical rotations students drew blood, counted white cells and platelets, stained whatever body fluid required examination, and worked up countless patients. When abused by unreasonable work demands, such as the requirement by one chief medical resident for their attendance on midnight rounds, the students had no recourse. This was not a time of student activism. A perceived bad attitude or unmet demand would jeopardize one's future success in the Match for internships. Interns and residents operated always at the brink of exhaustion, seeming to be on perpetual call. A shared vocabulary no longer spoke of individual patients but rather "the asthmatic" or "the Marfan's" or "the guy with tabes." Women younger than midlife were "girls" while young black men in that segregated hospital were "boys."

We began the process of wrapping our emotions tightly in the insulation of science and professional distance. In the tightly competitive environment students and housestaff alike feigned indifference to academic pressure and the opinions of superiors. No one ever spoke of how grief was to be addressed or bad news imparted. Never were the issues of health and well-being of medical students addressed. When President Kennedy was assassinated and I, and others, felt sorrow and loss, the attending physician on my ward warned us most sternly that we should not expect any time off on Monday to watch the televised funeral or participate in the national day of mourning. We were physicians-to-be and we were expected to be aloof from such considerations.

On a June day in 1964 we paraded to a podium to receive an ornate piece of paper from a university official who shook our hand but did not meet our gaze. The senior class of a year earlier had not been accorded even this recognition. The ceremony attested to our academic accomplishments. Our emotional competence was assumed.

THE GIRL IN THE
GLASS BOX

ᵈᵞᵖ

B.G. Williams lived in a glass box at Baltimore City Hospital. She was my first patient on my first clinical rotation, but B.G. had no awareness of this.

Her mother had come to the emergency room in advanced labor. She had not sought any prenatal care. Shortly after her uncomplicated labor and delivery, she disappeared into the night. The address on her registration forms was fictitious and efforts to locate her failed.

B.G. (for baby girl) had thick, curly black hair, dark brown skin, and all her external parts were fully formed. From the moment of her birth she was deeply cyanotic, which led to her immediate placement in a glass and steel isolette. B.G. Williams had but one ventricle in her heart.

On the second day of her life, B.G. became my charge. The first day of the initial clinical rotation is for the medical student a high moment, a mixture of anticipation and fear which we hope to camouflage. Several of us began our work on the pediatric service of this sister hospital of Johns Hopkins.

As we made initial morning rounds with the resident and intern we built our lists of patients whom we would most closely follow: a little girl permanently impaired by measles encephalitis, a thin six-year-old girl soon to die of acute leukemia, a boy paralyzed by polio. Two young black boys whose nervous systems had been devastated by lead poisoning from ingested paint flakes shared a corner of the ward, part of a detoxification study.

We paused at the isolette. "B.G. Williams," the name tag said.

"Not much hope here." The resident nodded toward me, and I began my list with a brief clinical summary of the bluish infant.

From my tiny charge I was to learn about the fluid, electrolyte, and nutritional needs of a newborn. I was to learn as well about cyanotic congenital heart disease. I was to learn how difficult is the placement of a tiny needle in the scalp vein of a child weighing not much more than my pediatrics textbook.

The team and the attending physician paused daily at B.G.'s glass box. Even in that oxygen rich environment, she was cyanotic, and with her attempts to cry her blueness deepened. The senior physician exemplified realistic empathy, which was the prevailing professional mood on that service.

"It can't be fixed," he said.

B.G. slipped further each day as her cyanosis intensified. I reviewed her numbers—vital signs, electrolytes, and hemoglobins—with the nurse who presided over the ward. In those shaky, uncertain days, there was happily always a nurse who probably did as much to support falsely bold medical students as she did for her pediatric patients.

"Too bad, it can't be fixed," she said.

My son had a name, a home, and parents who loved him and fretted when he had a cold or colic. He was 14 months old and was not cyanotic. He could cry and laugh and toddle at increasing speeds, until finally he toppled over or came to rest against a chair or table. My son could share his carriage space with a sack of groceries as his mother pushed both home from the Giant Food Store.

Somewhere in Baltimore B.G. Williams' mother had only the soreness of recent childbirth to remind her of a night's stay at Baltimore City Hospital. What did she feel as she left the hospital that night? Did she sense that her child had some fatal flaw? Did she care? Was she married? Was B.G. the result of careless lovemaking between chance acquaintances? Was this the woman's first pregnancy?

B.G.'s skin was purple. Her movements were weaker, and she seemed to spend much of her time sleeping. When she would screw up her face to cry, no sound came forth as she opened her mouth. I held her briefly each morning in my cupped hands.

Two weeks into her life she died. I was not present. On rounds the following morning her isolette was empty and cleaned and pushed against a wall. Her nurse explained to me that she had simply stopped breathing during the night. Later that day an autopsy confirmed the diagnosis of a single ventricle.

My son is 36 now, the eldest of four boys who were each given a name at birth. Each was taken home in his mother's arms to be nurtured and raised.

B.G. Williams had neither name nor home apart from a glass box in which she lived for 14 days. Without the cardiac anomaly, perhaps she would have made her way to an orphanage, and perhaps she would have been adopted by a couple who would have loved her dearly. Perhaps, a grandmother would have learned of her existence and come to the hospital to claim her. She would be 35 years old at this writing. Possibly, she would not have survived the poverty and violence which racked Baltimore's inner city neighborhoods. She might have found a teacher who took a special interest in her. Her writing might have shown promise and by hard work, steady application, and encouragement of her adoptive mother, she just might have graduated from high school and gone to college or found work in a store or a factory.

Back then, I could not comprehend this life that was not to be. I recall sadness and the awareness that I was expected to remain aloof from sentiment. I said a silent prayer for the soul of B.G. Williams. And our rounds continued.

CALORIES

AND ELECTROLYTES

Certain patients stand as landmarks in the same way as rings on the stump of an old oak tree. They document a stage, a finite piece of the past. Sally was such a growth ring for me.

She was in her late 60s and had come to Johns Hopkins Hospital with a painful belly. She had a perforated colon for which surgery was performed, but things went terribly wrong thereafter. Fistulous connections developed between loops of bowel and bowel and skin. In that pre-ICU day, Sally lived in a private room with private duty nurses in a building named for the famed surgeon, William Halsted. Her resident and intern visited each morning. Her care was my responsibility the rest of the time. I was a senior student serving my ten-week surgical rotation. No one told me that Sally's case was hopeless; weeks passed before I realized that she was dying.

She lived on a farm on Maryland's eastern shore. Her serene face belonged on a cover of *The Progressive Farmer* magazine. Her dark eyes never wavered from whomever she addressed. Weathered skin told of long hours in outside work, possibly tending a garden or helping her husband in the fields. Prominent cheekbones added to the firmness of her countenance. From the shoulders upward, those being the parts visible above the sheet's edge, she might have been anyone's healthy, smiling, and caring grandmother. She immediately reminded me of my own magical Aunt Mary Paul who lived on a Georgia farm. Sally spoke slowly and deliberately just as if she were in a store or social gathering rather than in the room of her impending death. She seemed oblivious to pain and the odor of pus and feces, which oozed into her dressings. She never acknowledged pain, only fatigue.

Every night she wore a nightcap. She did not like to be seen in the mornings until she was "fixed up." Her nurse combed out her long gray hair and helped arrange it into a large bun atop her head. The nurse applied her lipstick and facial powder. Sally called me "honey" and called her nurse by her surname.

There is a special type of nurse who, despite the most appalling clinical circumstances, maintains the ability to sustain compassionate care of the highest professional standard. The name of Sally's daytime nurse, with whom I worked most closely, has dropped from the tapes of my memory. She was not much younger than Sally. She had graying hair, cut short and topped by the cap that all nurses wore as a badge of honor. Whenever I entered Sally's room the nurse, if seated, stood to greet me. She succinctly reviewed the events since my last visit and we studied the clinical graphs. She timed changes of dressings to coincide with my early morning visit. Sally's bluish abdomen bulged and was dotted with fistulae draining foul fluids. Ever so gently the nurse cleaned the skin and applied fresh bulky gauze dressings, a routine to be repeated several times each shift. Only when Sally slept did the nurse seem relaxed. Otherwise she tended to her patient's every need, washing her face, fluffing her pillow, and raising a glass of water to her lips. I wanted to ask her how she did it, how she could manage a smile and confer gentle strength to Sally in such a hopeless setting. Nurses on teaching wards are cut from special cloth.

On daily rounds, which followed my early morning visit, our clinical team paused to study the charted measurements of Sally's waning life. I offered a brief review of the past day. Her abdomen was not examined. Sometimes a perfunctory inquiry was directed at the patient or nurse before we moved to the next patient.

Sally's nurse knew more than I about what was going on and what needed to be done for the care of her patient. Ever the diplomat, when I made a miscalculation or suggested a wrong-headed wrinkle to therapy, she knew how to guide therapy back to a stable track. She led unobtrusively.

There were fevers and cultures and antibiotics. After a while there were resistant bacteria and yeast everywhere. I dreaded going into Sally's room. I had to maintain "the mask," a screen that physicians must learn to hold up so that the patient cannot sense our inner despair or pessimism. The foul odor of hopelessly infected flesh intensified and extended beyond the closed door with its curtained window. Any passerby could sense that death was close.

One day, I dropped my guard in a conversation with a senior resident.

"I'm having a tough time with Sally," I said.

"If you can't stand the heat, you don't belong in the kitchen," the resident replied.

The code was re-emphasized. "Keep your feelings to yourself." Better still, you should bury your feelings or pretend that they do not exist.

Slowly, Sally's tissues broke down. Her face became drawn, her eyes hollow, and her speech thin and raspy. She still managed a smile and extended her hand to mine in greeting. After altering the day's calories and electrolytes, the nurse and I faced each other across the head of Sally's bed encouraging our patient's reminiscences of sunny days and hard work. Most of her people were dead. I never encountered a visitor. She asked that we pray for her.

Sally clung to life on the last day of my ten-week rotation on the Hopkins surgical service. She was gaunt and jaundiced and too weak to lift her head from her pillow. Her hair was still beautifully combed and her makeup artistically applied. Her voice was now a whisper. I told her I would drop by to see her whenever I had a chance. She thanked me. Outside the room, I thanked the nurse and shook her hand. I finally asked how on earth she could perform such work day after day. She said it was simply her job. For a moment, her eyes glistened with tears. She thanked me, and we parted.

"Should have," and "meant to," but several days passed before I returned to that surgical ward. Another patient resided in Sally's room.

At the nursing station they told me of her death less than a week after my rotation ended. I never saw the private duty nurse again. I wanted to write to her, but I had no address. Some duty or deadline quickly called me from that ward. Perhaps I was afraid to linger.

I cared for Sally for ten weeks in 1964. Perhaps in a time of better antibiotics and nutritional support she would have had a chance at survival, but I think not. There were simply too many drainage ports, and each day brought a fresh one. The technical legacy of those two women was that thereafter I could rapidly calculate fluid, electrolyte, and caloric needs for any patient. But I see now that Sally and her nurse were sisters, not biological but spiritual, who had staked out a lonely, disease-corrupted corner of this earth to make a stand. Neither would allow the other to surrender to the awfulness that surrounded them. They stood for beauty and graciousness and for the responsibility of teaching powerful lessons to a medical student who wandered in one day.

DON'T DARE MISS

To earn needed money I worked in the Hopkins blood bank two weekends each month. I was called a "donor room assistant." Today, I would be called a "phlebotomist." My job was to obtain a pint of blood from the donors who appeared on Saturdays and Sundays. We maintained our own roster of potential donors categorized by blood types. These were my favorite clients because they were familiar with the process of blood donation and could remain relaxed throughout. They also had large dependable peripheral veins.

Other donors came from the streets. Some wanted to donate blood for a friend or family member who had recently been injured. A few donors were lured by promises of payment for their blood. I sensed that this money was not destined for educational or household purposes.

As part-time jobs went at the hospital, this one was not bad. I earned ten dollars an hour, my highest rate of pay up to that time. Frequently, a donor recounted the surgery or hardship of his family member or friend for whom the blood was destined. Most of the time I could impale an arm vein on the first attempt. After a while I was almost cocky. My routine was flawless as I motioned each donor to lie down and trust me. After a quick reconnaissance for the best vein I applied my tourniquet, cleaned the overlying skin, punctured the vein, and sat back as the bottle filled with blood.

One Sunday afternoon I faced my maximal challenge. A large African American man, who looked as if he could step at that very moment into the offensive line of the Baltimore Colts, arrived to donate blood. He was a little bit drunk and more than a little bit angry. His brother-in-law had been shot and he was here at his wife's insistence to give blood. The potential for violence accompanied him. Turning him down because he was inebriated was not an option. I felt that he would demolish the donor room and probably kill me as well. His huge body overhung the narrow stretcher for donors. His arms resembled those of the legendary Cincinnati Reds slugger Ted Kluszewski. I applied the tourniquet and swabbed his mid-arm with alcohol. There were simply no veins to be seen or felt anywhere. His massive muscular arms must have drawn their blood supply from subterranean vessels.

He stared at me. "Don't dare miss," he said.

I checked the other arm. Again nothing. He became more impatient as I placed his hand in a pan of warm water. Usually this would stimulate blood flow which in turn would highlight a vein. All I needed was a single vein which would accommodate my 14-gauge needle in a quick and painless thrust.

He glowered. His growing impatience was palpable. Then I noted a small vein just above the elbow on the posterior aspect of one arm. I could not reach it if he lay supine. For the only time in my two-year career as phlebotomist I moved the donor to a chair. I applied the tourniquet high on his upper arm while he rested his forearm on his lap. I did not know if the vein represented a mirage or an answer to prayer. He flinched slightly as I pushed the needle into his treelike arm. Nothing. I wiggled the needle and advanced it further. Still nothing. And then, like some sort of hematologic manna, the plastic tubing to the citrated bottle began to fill ever so slowly with a column of maroon liquid, which slowly advanced until it dripped into the bottle. I did not dare move the needle or tape it down. Instead, I held it at a 90° angle as the bottle slowly filled.

A coworker from the lab came through at that moment, scoped the scene, and asked, "What in the hell are you doing?"

"I'm drawing blood," I said.

I did, and I survived. I did not know who eventually received this unit of blood. We lacked testing for any infectious disease save syphilis, so any of our pints of blood had the potential for mayhem. The patient, for his part, continued to grumble as he waited out the obligatory few minutes before release from the blood bank. The promise of violence was never fulfilled, at least in the Hopkins blood bank. Woe to anyone who might have offended him after he departed the hospital that afternoon.

THE CRY

During internship she killed herself, slashing her wrists weeks after beginning her housestaff job in another city. Although we shared several rotations during medical school, I never felt that I knew her especially well. I respected her and grieved her loss.

She was a demure, blue-eyed presence, the type of person who seems to add a certain stability to any group. She smiled softly at the jokes of others but initiated none of her own. She seldom spoke and never volunteered answers during clinical rounds. When asked a direct question, she invariably had a correct succinct answer. When those of us on her clinical rotations complained or expressed paranoia, she seemed unperturbed, her countenance varying from neutral to half-smiling.

If she encountered difficulties with a patient or her studies, she showed no evidence. Her oral presentations of patients to the attending physician showed a wide range and command of recent clinical literature. Our resident complained that her written work-ups were far too long, easily doubling the five or six typed pages that we would submit. Once when her left wrist was extended beyond the cuff of her white lab coat, I noticed an irregular, white scar where her watchband usually circled. I wondered about this.

During a shared surgical rotation, it was her time to present a case to a professor known for his general disdain for medical students. This aging eminence prided himself on toughness toward all of his subordinates. Most of our professors and instructors, while demanding, were civil and generally supportive of our publicly enunciated work. There were, however, scattered through all clinical departments, predatory faculty whose goal was the humiliation of medical students and the terrorization of housestaff. They behaved as hyenas on the scent of a wounded antelope.

My own exposure to this ordeal occurred at surgical grand rounds where I presented a case of complicated appendicitis to a young assistant professor. He repeatedly interrupted my monologue, derided my observations, then began to question me closely about the life and death of Harry Houdini. Luckily, I knew of Houdini's presumed death from a ruptured appendix and could thereby parry some of his verbal blows. Nevertheless, this was vile psychological hazing from a faculty member who demeaned his position of authority. I could only grin and store my anger.

My colleague's presentation began quietly, but after a couple of minutes the professor interrupted her. He asked several questions, not all of them relevant. He motioned for her to continue only to interrupt her again and challenge her skills at history taking. He belittled her examination and peppered her with questions about the physicians whose names were attached to clinical syndromes. She blinked hard. Her eyes moistened and then reddened. The surgeon did not relent. His tone was biting, then outright insulting. She stammered but continued. He stood, looming, as the giant might have intimidated Jack atop the beanstalk. Her voice faltered repeatedly as she tried to finish. Insult followed insult, and a tear spilled down her cheek from eyes now frightened.

Finally, she finished and could take her seat, dejectedly, while the surgeon continued his rumbling diatribe. She was wounded, but by the following day she was back to her usual quiet, stable demeanor.

She matched for a prestigious internship in another city. In the remaining weeks of our senior year she remained a modest, knowledgeable colleague. Occasionally, grayish rims beneath her eyes suggested a burden of fatigue.

Though many of us were vulnerable in that medical school of high stress and high reputation, most of us could retreat either to our families or to circles of beer-drinking or bridge-playing friends. We could play with our children or find a pick-up game of touch football to blow off our ire and stress. She apparently had no such blessing or resource.

Upon the 25th anniversary of the graduation of my class, I received multiple letters of invitation to commemorative celebration. I received additional letters soliciting cash donations. I dusted off the picture of our white clad senior class standing on the steps of the medical school library. I searched faces, trying to recall names and to answer the question "Whatever became of ... ?" My eyes were drawn to the front row, to the young woman, elegant and outwardly unruffled with a gentle half smile. Her career was never to be because of a cry not uttered or not heard by the rest of us.

NASHVILLE

1964~1968, 1971

As a boy, on Saturday nights I station-surfed on my plastic-encased Silvertone radio. I could easily pick up the Grand Ole Opry broadcast live from Ryman Auditorium in Nashville, Tennessee, on "50-thousand-watt, clear-channel WSM." The nasally intoned lyrics told of lonely nights and lost loves, life in the saddle, and longings for home. Fiddles, guitars, three-fingered banjos, and mandolins accompanied the singers. A musical amalgam of country, gospel, western, and bluegrass mingled with commercials and Minnie Pearl's monologues of life in Grinder's Switch. For many families in the South, Saturday nights were organized around these radiocasts. Bill Monroe, Lester Flatt, Earl Scruggs—all were household names among the far-flung audience. This was the Voice of America for Americans. When Little Jimmy Dickens of the Opry came to the stage of the LaGrange Theater, we felt that we had reached the upper echelon of entertainment.

Twenty years later I sat in Nashville's Centennial Park at a concert featuring Mother Maybelle Carter, her autoharp, and her three daughters. The melodies and lyrics had not changed but country music, once a stepchild, was now a major business generating mansions and studios and huge stores hawking records and autographed paraphernalia of the stars. Songwriters, singers, and instrumentalists flocked to the city, some to fame, most to continued oblivion. Cars and buses from throughout the Southeast and Midwest streamed into town each weekend to attend those Saturday evening performances. Country music was soon to generate a vast new Opryland complex where a sleek, huge auditorium would host an upscale Opry. The lovelorn of the lyrics were now more likely to ride into the sunset of loneliness in their pickup trucks than on horseback.

In sharp contrast to the jeans-clad denizens of the music world, Nashville's wearers of business suits accurately foresaw another boom in the city's business and financial enterprises. The self-satisfied city of the Old South, where politicians named "Big Evil" and "Little Evil" had once held sway, was ready to go places even if it knew not quite where.

There was still the matter of racism to be solved, as a nasty sit-in at a whites-only Morrison's Cafeteria demonstrated. A highly vocal confrontation on the Vanderbilt campus demanded desegregation of that university's school of divinity. A huge economic chasm further divided the races.

Similar divisions existed in Nashville's medical community. The city was home to affluent, all-white Vanderbilt Medical School and impoverished all-black Meharry Medical College. Vanderbilt boasted a growing endowment, an active research faculty, and fiefdoms over which presided the region's top medical specialists. Meharry, founded in 1876, struggled to stay open while training the majority of the nation's African American physicians.

A handful of Nashville's white physicians worked to maintain a frail bridge between the two institutions, providing lectures, clinical teaching, and attending services for the Meharry students. As a consequence of these efforts two Meharry students requested a clinical rotation on Vanderbilt's clinical research unit in 1967. Assuming the request had cleared all the necessary administrative hurdles, in my role as chief medical resident I finalized the arrangements. One Monday morning the two students began work. Hardly had they set foot on the research unit than the attending physician summoned me to his office and launched against me the most blistering diatribe I had ever sustained. He repeatedly referred to the Meharry students as "those people"; they were lambasted in absentia. Shaken and fearing that my next job would be as an orderly in some rural hospital, I retreated to the office of my boss, the departmental chairman. Tall and handsome, he was in his early 30s when he had moved to the chair of medicine from New York. The young faculty that he recruited would take the institution to a new level of national respect during his tenure.

After hearing me out, my boss phoned the irate research chief, a man much his senior, and ever so calmly indicated that the Meharry students were there at his personal invitation. He was certain that the chief would make every possible effort to ensure both their welcome and their full participation in departmental activities. Their clerkship proceeded uneventfully. One of the students later worked with distinction as a clinical fellow in Vanderbilt's division of endocrinology.

Of such small acts, justice is born.

THAT'S ALL

&

Joe arrived on the ward mid-afternoon. He had been admitted from
the medical clinic following detection of a large cavity in the apex of
his right lung. This tall and muscular African American raised tobacco
west of Nashville. Because of progressive weakness, fever, and a worsening cough, he had traveled to Nashville for medical evaluation. His
examination confirmed recent weight loss. Breath sounds over his
right upper chest were diminished and rasping. He had to get well in a
hurry so that his current crop would be properly harvested.

Conveniently, Joe coughed up a wad of grayish-yellow mucus,
which I took to the lab for microscopic examination. The lot of the
intern in 1964 was to perform all laboratory tests, except blood
chemistries. I expected to find acid-fast organisms of tuberculosis.

For the only time in my career I saw tiny yellow "sulfur granules"
in his sputum. Under the microscope the yellow dots became tangles
of gram positive bacilli. Joe suffered from actinomycosis.

Certain diseases, despite their rare occurrence, are highlighted repeatedly throughout medical training. These are the "zebras," exotic
diseases which, once diagnosed, give the medical detective special
bragging rights. Porphyrias, Wilson's disease, thymoma—such are the
uncommon ailments that lead us along circuitous and often quite ex-

pensive diagnostic pathways. Actinomycosis is one such entity. From earliest days in microbiology this diagnosis was placed in the memory loop reserved for special maladies. "Sulfur granules" were guaranteed an appearance on final examinations in microbiology, although few of us would ever see them outside the teaching lab. Joe's sputum created a special moment.

I called my resident. This was a new observation for him. Other housestaff were called to peer down the microscope. We had before us the microbiological equivalent of moon dust. I alerted the head of the infectious disease service, and he confirmed our diagnosis.

A covey of young house officers and clinical fellows followed the chief as we walked briskly to Joe's bedside. We anticipated a definitive teaching experience, which would establish a link between an oddity of basic science and an actual patient. Perhaps our names would be attached in some way to the inevitable clinical paper.

The patient's bed was empty. His personal belongings were nowhere to be seen. The other patients in his four-bed ward reported that Joe had departed for home. One of the roommates reported that Joe had been taken by wheelchair to the x-ray department for further studies of his pulmonary lesion. Upon completing the x-rays the technician had said, "That will be all." To Joe this indicated that his brief hospital stay was completed. He returned to his room, discussed the encounter with his fellow patients, packed his bag, and left for parts unknown.

"Find him!" the chief said.

The admission sheet listed a Star Route address in a county in western Tennessee.

Over subsequent days my resident and I contacted public health officials and the sheriff's department in that county. We consulted telephone operators, but no number for Joe existed. Our patient could not be located. Finally, we gave up. Perhaps actinomycosis really did not exist, and Joe had been a mirage. We supposed that his lung infection would likely worsen, thereby prompting his return to our medical clinic. But he never came back. We directed our efforts toward the more mundane diseases that came our way, continuing the house officer's traditional quest for a reportable case. From time to time during the next few weeks Joe's name came up at morning report. Then with the press of other duties, we forgot about him.

Six years later I worked my weekly assignment in the Vanderbilt Clinic, this time as a postgraduate fellow. As I scanned the names of patients to be seen that afternoon, Joe's name leapt out at me. I turned to scan the faces in the lobby. I recognized the tall farmer immediately. Except for being somewhat heavier, he had not visibly aged since our earlier meeting. He appeared quite healthy. I greeted him and ushered him to an examination room ahead of his scheduled time.

He told me that he felt quite well and that he farmed full time. Had a public health nurse not detected high blood pressure at a health fair, he would not have come to the clinic this day.

I examined his chest. Nothing. I ordered a chest x-ray. The thinnest wisp of scar tissue extended toward the apex of his right lung. There was no evidence of any active pulmonary disease.

"Tell me what happened," I said.

Following his presumed dismissal from Vanderbilt Hospital, Joe returned home to a farm located on a remote, unpaved, back road. Because of his continued cough, he consulted a family practitioner in a nearby community.

"And what did he do?" I asked.

The family physician examined him but did not obtain a chest x-ray. Nor did he check any laboratory studies. He prescribed "some pills," which Joe faithfully took for several weeks. As his strength returned, he resumed work on his farm. He again felt strong and happy. His blood pressure, elevated when measured at the recent health fair, was now normal. I reassured Joe that his health was robust. We shook hands to conclude his second visit to the Vanderbilt Clinic.

AT THE VA

⌾ϱ

Nashville's sparkling new Veterans Administration Hospital at the edge of the Vanderbilt campus was perpetually full. This was assured by a lengthy waiting list of patients, an x-ray department that moved with glacial slowness—never more than four barium procedures per day—and a policy of prohibiting the dismissal of a patient until a replacement was on his way to the ward.

Despite a staff of talented faculty and physicians, we interns became progressively cynical as we served our clinical rotations at the VA. There were relatively few veterans of actual combat. Many illnesses on the medical service stemmed from self-neglect and abuse rather than the effects of military service. Alcoholism in all of its complex forms, diseases related to incessant smoking, and social destitution were common reasons for admission. Some veterans had become quite expert in manipulating the VA's administrative system to prolong their hospitalizations and thereby enhance their disability pensions. Veterans of World War I and a rare veteran or two of the Spanish American War were granted automatic admission. Older veterans sometimes sought admission as they migrated in the autumn of the year to warmer Florida weather. Nashville was a convenient stopover. The medical clinic stayed full of downcast men for whom mandatory participation in military service seemed to be the only highlight in lives of frustration and economic struggle. Later experience taught us that these sad men were veterans by coincidence and their military service had little to do with smoldering disappointments. For some veterans camaraderie with their peers and the VA staff seemed to represent the only social structure in their lives. Sometimes older veterans seemed ashamed that they had to rely on a government hospital for their care at a time of illness.

One early patient was different. He was slender, 40ish, and a lieutenant colonel in the U.S. Army. While serving with a group of advisors in South Vietnam, he had sustained a myocardial infarction subsequently complicated by a stroke. I never knew why he was not sent to an Army hospital for his convalescence. I never saw a visitor at his bedside. He knew that this illness meant the end of his military career and that he was unlikely ever to be well enough to work in any situation.

I knew vaguely that South Vietnam was a part of former French Indochina. The colonel described a nation torn by civil war in which a small group of Americans advised the side friendly to the West. Many on this side were Roman Catholic, fierce opponents of the Communist insurgents who were supported by North Vietnam. Fighting consisted of brutal attacks in the jungle in which the enemy—he used the term "Vietcong," which I heard for the first time—quickly faded away. He predicted a long and nasty war. One day, his bed was empty. I did not know his next destination.

Further along the same ward one of the great heroes of World War I, a Medal of Honor awardee, struggled through his final days of severe and progressive vascular disease. This was the giant in final disrepair. He was insensate, incontinent, and severely bent by arthritis. Family members stayed with him continually in his private room. His medical records constituted the highest stack on the ward, promising an administrative nightmare for the unlucky resident who would someday have to dictate a death summary. The hero died days after I moved to my next assignment.

Having built models of most American fighter aircraft of World War II, I was drawn to a 50-year-old man who had been admitted for alcoholism and cirrhosis. From his history I learned that he had flown P-38s in combat in the Pacific Theater. The model of the shiny twin engine fighter had been my favorite to build. I had read extensively about the airplane and its exploits. As my patient improved, I sought further details. What was the aircraft like? How did the plane handle? He recollected little. Did he not remember? Had alcohol eroded his ability to remember? Did it hurt to remember?

Gradually, as our shared time on the ward progressed, we found a common, comfortable language. Fear and exhaustion stood out in his memory. One day he spoke of the stimulant pills that he took to maintain alertness as he flew his missions. At night he relied on alcohol to relax him and to induce sleep. Many in his squadron were killed, and new pilots joined his squadron weekly. After the war he was never able to shake his dependence on "diet pills" and whiskey. He could neither stay married nor hold a job for very long. He had a partial disability pension for psychological reasons. He felt that his health was broken. Already, he had survived two major gastrointestinal hemorrhages. He acknowledged that, once released from hospitalization, he would not be able to refrain from alcohol. After a few weeks he was transferred to a VA convalescent facility.

Years later I cared for two other World War II veterans of combat flight who described similar experiences of titrating "uppers" and "downers" in dealing with the extreme stress of their missions. Their wondrous silver machines exceeded levels of human emotional tolerance. I learned from these veterans that some wounds of war leave no visible scars. Sometimes the stresses of battle would not manifest themselves until years after military service.

Our penchant as physicians to categorize patients neatly as "alcoholics" or "personality disorders" robs our patients of their human identity and us of the opportunity to understand the real causes of their illnesses. Even 20 and 30 years after fighting, the fear and loneliness in the pilots' stories were palpable. Too easily we neglect the humanity of our patients, covering it with a tarpaulin of a disease entity.

In 1965 the Nashville VA acquired its first dialysis machine: a gray, steel, tub-like device. The director of this fledgling unit was dubbed "The Earl of Tubs." Because there were far more patients with chronic renal failure than there would be slots for life-sustaining dialytic treatment, the VA devised a mechanism to establish priorities for therapy. Uremic veterans were scheduled for interviews in which the "social worth" of each man would be assessed on a convoluted scale. Presumably, felons and drug addicts would remain under the traditional inadequate therapy of diet and medication. The chosen ones would have their blood regularly cleansed in anticipation of eventual renal transplantation.

One particular patient had caused teams of housestaff more grief than his peers. He had chronic renal failure. He was consistently unable, or unwilling, to take his medication and to follow any semblance of a renal diet. Frequently, he appeared in the admitting office inebriated and in a rumpled and unshaven state. He did not hesitate to unload a string of oaths upon his intern and resident. Oftentimes he signed out of the hospital before treatment could be completed. He personified the difficult patient.

Then came the transformation. The process for prioritization for the dialysis program had been widely publicized. On the day of his interview, the previously disheveled veteran appeared in a dapper white Palm Beach suit and new straw hat. He carried a large Bible with a white cover embossed in gold. He was quite confident of his chances as he visited his former habitat on the ward. He declared that he was a new man, he had found Jesus, and he regularly attended church. He no longer needed alcohol. He thanked us profusely for his earlier care. He was not among the chosen.

Military service in a time of war is the toughest demand our nation places on its citizens. In World War II almost all of my community's healthy men under age 35 either volunteered or were drafted, usually into the Army. Many would be recalled to duty during the Korean War. With succeeding decades the burden of service fell progressively on those lacking the political connections, the money, or the academic grades to gain exemption from the military draft.

The VA rotations showed me a side of military service far removed from the heroics reported in military dispatches or on the movie screen. These were men who had typically lost two to four years from civilian pursuits. Some had borne the constant dangers and fears of front line combat. Many others had driven trucks or constructed roads, barracks, or airfields, or performed the countless tedious duties of sustaining an army in the field and fleet at sea. Boring routines and cheap alcohol had facilitated ruinous habits for many men stuck in strange places. The VA medical system, imperfect and administratively burdened, represented a safety net which ensured, if nothing else, a high standard of medical care for former soldiers, sailors, and airmen.

The great majority of the one-time volunteers and draftees in the Nashville VA hospital of the 1960s would have preferred to remain at home pursuing a livelihood, marrying, and creating families. After World War II and the Korean War most veterans returned to full-time civilian roles. Some veterans never regained momentum or opportunity to proceed with life. All of these men had for a time, whether grumbling, afraid, impatient, or fired with patriotic zeal, kept me safe as I grew through boyhood. I respect them.

SHOCK THERAPY

He was a farmer from middle Tennessee, a slightly built man whose chronically tanned and weathered skin spoke of endless days in his fields and pastures. He grew corn and soybeans and tended a small herd of cattle. His wiry frame carried no fat. He could have been any age from 30 to 60. He had few teeth, barely anchored by his receding gums. His fractured grammar documented an early end to his formal education. He was admitted to Vanderbilt Hospital because of severe rheumatoid arthritis.

This was the first hospitalization of his 30-odd years. He recalled childhood fractures and lacerations treated as an outpatient. Arthritis involving his hands, elbows, and knees had begun explosively a few years earlier. He had consulted nearby physicians and chiropractors in a search for relief.

The pain and swelling in his hands and wrists made the daily chores on his farm all but impossible. His wife and children pitched in to maintain the farm's viability. Recently, he had discovered methods to reduce the unremitting pain.

Despite the years of active arthritis with ongoing pain, his fingers, hands, and wrists showed remarkable ranges of movement. He exhibited few of the severe joint deformities so characteristic of his disease.

My resident and I performed all of the appropriate medical center tests, which confirmed the diagnosis of quite severe rheumatoid arthritis. Our consultant in rheumatology expressed surprise at the farmer's supple fingers and wrists. Following our bedside conference with the attending physician we outlined to the patient a program of physical therapy, daily high doses of aspirin, and weekly injection of gold salts. I inquired how he had maintained such surprising use of his hands despite aggressive disease. His treatment method follows.

Disillusioned by the inability of any medical practitioner to relieve the pain and swelling of his joints, the farmer had devised his own treatment protocol. With the help of his wife, he fashioned and applied splints to his hands and wrists each evening at bedtime. His wife first taped his fingers to a thick piece of plywood. She then pressed a second slab against the dorsum of each hand and wrist while she tightened C-clamps until the joints were fully extended between the wooden rectangles. He slept with his hands thus flattened. This routine was repeated nightly.

One evening, while working in his barn, the farmer suffered a brief accidental shock while working on his ancient tractor. This seemed to relieve the pain of arthritis for several days. He then invented a second therapeutic regimen. Each evening, while he stood on damp burlap bags, he grasped spark plug wires on his tractor. When his wife turned the ignition key, the resulting shock would throw him backward to the ground. The "shock therapy" was repeated nightly. He assured me that the shock relieved his pain more effectively than any medication. In fact, he took no analgesics of any kind. Had his brother-in-law not insisted that he seek medical consultation at Vanderbilt, the farmer would have remained contentedly home caring for his crops and cattle, entrusting further improvement to his home remedies.

A day later, he announced that he must return home to attend to his work. He did not wish to offend us or to denigrate our recommendations in any way. "Buddy, I just don't cotton after that," he apologized to me.

I assume his tractor was cranked later that day as he held firmly to the engine's wires.

Folk medicine abounds in the South. Some practices may be quite distinct for an individual or within a family. Other customs are more widely dispersed.

In elementary school my classmate Jasper pulled up the leg of his overalls to show a wondrous, irregular black scar on his thigh. He had fallen from a car fender, slashing his leg on a metallic license plate. His mother sprinted into his house, reached into a chimney, and pulled down a handful of soot. This she immediately applied to Jasper's wound, which she then bandaged tightly. Even in this modern day I see an occasional elderly patient with a deeply pigmented scar. When the circumstances of the injury can be recalled, the technique of soot application is reconfirmed. Perhaps sulfur or some other element in the soot sterilized the torn flesh and prevented subsequent infection.

Copper bracelets remain in wide use as a prevention or therapy for arthritis. In my childhood, thin copper wire bracelets or anklets were worn by adults and children on the farms and in the mill villages. To-day, the copper is more often fashioned into elaborate bracelets. El-derly patients recall copper bracelets worn by their grandparents. If the copper wearer has never experienced arthritis, then the orange metal is venerated for its preventive properties. When inflamed joints antedate the wearing of copper jewelry, healing properties are attributed to the new bodily adornments.

More recently, raisin and gin therapy have been added to the arsenal of home nostrums for arthritis. Even the most teetotaling, elderly pa-tients tell me that gin-soaked raisins have done wonders for their painful joints. The recipe? A box of raisins is dumped into a bowl containing a quart of gin, and the mixture is allowed to age for several days. Depend-ing on the severity of joint pain, 12 to 20 of the gin-bloated raisins are eaten daily or two to three times daily if the pain is not quickly abated.

I listen. I do not laugh. The various remedies are invested with weighty family tradition and the full power of placebo therapy. If a home treatment protocol seems dangerous or toxic, such as the taking of small amounts of turpentine in the treatment of colds, I discourage it. I doubt that the farmer with rheumatoid arthritis could have been dissuaded from using his electrotherapy. Certainly, therapy for rheumatoid arthritis as it existed in 1964 might not have improved the functional status of his hands. Given the uneven and, at times, accidental progression of medical therapeutics, scientific rationales for spark plug wires and alcohol-laden raisins may yet be determined. In the mean time, I will continue to listen.

FOOLS RUSH IN

I was chief resident for the Vanderbilt medical service. The year represented the icing on the cake of housestaff experience. This curious and hectic job blended elements of foreman, shop steward, medical consultant, schedule maker, flak catcher, and general problem solver. I had not anticipated the additional role of personal physician for residents and their spouses.

A highly competent assistant resident became terrified when he experienced a painful, purulent urethral discharge. He concealed the symptoms for days, fearing disgrace as a culture labeled with his name proceeded through the bacteriologic lab. He reasoned that if he simply ignored his symptoms, they might disappear. We concocted an alias for all of the appropriate cultures and serology. His illness quickly resolved following tetracycline therapy.

More serious was the fulminant hepatitis suffered by another resident. He became progressively jaundiced and his liver enzyme values soared. The best efforts of a bevy of consultants failed. Therapy with high doses of corticosteroids was quite controversial then, and we were hesitant to employ it. We young physicians, capable of treating almost casually the most acute and complicated of illnesses, caught glimpses of our mortality as one of our own struggled to recover. In a bedside conference with the chiefs of medicine and gastroenterology we elected an aggressive trial of steroid therapy. I tried to convey confidence as I explained this decision to our ill colleague who reminded me that we had his trust. Within days the crisis of his illness had passed, and we breathed a collective sigh of relief and thanksgiving.

The clinical rotation for another house officer was not going well. He seemed distracted, his conversation mechanical. The attending physician on his service called me to express his concern. The senior physician had inquired of the resident if the resident were ill or if there were problems. The physician had been assured there were none. Other residents on his team sensed that these were tough times for him and, like members of a military platoon, tried to provide some extra coverage and help.

Before I left the hospital that evening I searched for him. He was not on call that evening. I was told that he had already departed for his apartment. I remained vaguely uneasy as I returned home, and so I telephoned after supper. He answered after a few rings. In response to my questions he reported that he was fine, just a little tired and that I should not worry. His monotone voice sounded detached.

I could not shake my rising apprehension. After an hour or so I drove to his apartment. There was no answer to the bell. The door was unlocked, and I entered. He stood in half light clad in shorts, holding a knife in one hand while blood dripped from the other wrist.

When I am frightened I have trouble speaking, and this was such an instance. I eased into the room, trying to keep a quaver from my voice. I had trouble catching my breath. I was aware of sweating profusely.

"Put it down," I told him.

"I can't go on," he said.

"Put the knife down," I said.

"There's no point," he answered.

I advanced hesitantly. He retreated a step or two.

"Stay back," he warned.

"Put the knife down," I repeated.

We circled the room. I did not know what to do. My voice was hoarse and strained. I felt physically drained and emotionally at the edge of panic. This situation was not described in any medical text. I talked nonstop, about what I do not remember, perhaps trying to calm myself as much as the injured physician. I talked and talked. I told him I would not leave. He spoke of overwhelming sadness. He could not continue to work as a physician. And, besides, with this act he knew that his career was at an end.

He agreed to sit, but he refused to consider hospitalization. If he went to Vanderbilt's emergency room, everyone would know of his self-inflicted injury. He would not permit me to call an ambulance or a relative. I continued to talk. Finally, he placed the knife on a tabletop.

We negotiated a plan. I would drive him to a nearby private hospital where no one need know either his identity or the circumstances of his injury. He agreed to let me call a physician on the staff at that hospital under whose name he would be admitted. I wrapped his wrist in a towel and pulled a raincoat over his shoulders.

The short drive to the hospital was quiet; he said nothing. I wanted the trip to be over. What if he should try to jump from my moving car? Finally, we reached the emergency room. Once inside, he refused help from a surgeon. I was the only person allowed to examine his wounds. With the help of one of the great prototypic ER nurses who know all of the proper procedures for helping the injured, I cleaned his wounds, jagged superficial gougings that fortunately had damaged neither tendon nor artery I had last sutured simple lacerations four years earlier during a surgical rotation in medical school.

"You'll want to use 4-0, won't you?" asked the nurse.

While she selected a local anesthetic and suture material, I sought to steady both my hands and my voice. Our patient lay quietly on the stretcher during the whole procedure. After what surely was one of the longest suturing efforts on record, the gashes were closed. I completed the admission paperwork. My night was over.

Eventually, the resident returned to work. Courageously, he acknowledged to his fellow residents how he had faced thoughts of suicide. He completed that year and the subsequent years of postgraduate training. I hope he happily practices to this day.

In housestaff training of those days, and I suspect it's the same for residents even today, we thought of ourselves as tough and self-contained physicians. We stored our grief, our hurt, and our anger like electrical capacitors ever at risk of sudden and unexpected discharge. We joked a lot and talked, but only to a point, afraid to show too much, afraid that a fellow resident or attending physician might sense that we were somehow too weak or emotionally brittle ever to be full-fledged physicians.

Throughout my years of professional training, no professor or counselor ever spoke to us of our own vulnerabilities. Perhaps it was assumed that we would absorb such insights as we dealt with our patients. A faculty member might stage a dinner or picnic for his team of residents or students. Maybe this was a veiled invitation for personal counsel if we should ever feel such a need.

Sometimes a rumor would circulate regarding a clinical clerk or intern who required a leave of absence because of disabling symptoms of stress. But because we lacked the emotional vocabulary to frame our own fears and hurts, how could we know how to reach out to wounded colleagues? We felt empathy; at the same time, we looked slightly askance. Patients sought our guidance. We crafted our own.

Unresolved personal stresses may be suppressed for a time by the demands of a busy schedule. Fatigue and exasperation undo this tidy separation of emotional compartments. Sometimes the result is an angry outburst delivered at the closest target, even if it's an unsuspecting loved one. Sometimes, alcohol is used to quiet the roil of emotion. Other times, the torpor of depression takes over.

I think of that night from time to time. Fools rush in because sometimes we have no choice.

LIGHTING UP

∂ϕ

Medical residents at Vanderbilt spent portions of each year on two-month rotations of various medical subspecialties. On some tours a resident might have little role beyond the performance of histories and physical examinations, which would be reported up the chain of academic command. Actual physical contact with a patient lessened at each successive level: resident, fellow, junior faculty, attending guru. At the appointed hour each afternoon the subspecialty phalanx set out with its chief in the vanguard. At each bedside stop the resident presented the details that related to the clinical problem of primary interest to the group. Questions were asked, sometimes of the patient. Comments were exchanged. The chief spoke, and we moved on.

The hematology service represented an alternative characterized by more soulful concern for each of the patients under its wing. A patient with leukemia was inseparable from the smear of her blood or bone marrow. No judgments were decreed on the basis of seniority. The heme team argued, disagreed, questioned, reflected. Although responsibility for leading the clinical service alternated among hematology faculty, everyone contributed to the animated discussions of the patients and their illnesses. Both in the clinic and in the hospital, contacts with patients and their families were intense, personal, and heartfelt.

Clyde was well known to the housestaff. The sinewy young farmer came to the clinic frequently and, in recent months, had required several hospitalizations because of multiple myeloma, which had become increasingly refractory to therapy. Usually the tanned, friendly man was accompanied by his wife. Next to his family and farming, Clyde loved hunting. He inspired immediate friendliness in everyone he met. Some weeks earlier, two members of the hematology staff had accepted Clyde's invitation to go quail hunting on his property. The physicians knew of the extensive skeletal damage inflicted by myeloma upon their patient and friend. They worried throughout the hunt that the recoil from Clyde's shotgun would shatter the bones of his arms and shoulders. The outing ended without injury.

I knew Clyde from a previous admission to the medical ward on which I worked and had been present at conferences in which his case launched discussions of plasma cells and multiple myeloma. As the resident on the hematology service I was to assist in the management of his final hospitalization.

Clyde arrived at the emergency room by ambulance. His terrified wife had called. Clyde had sneezed. Severe pain immediately developed in his neck and for a brief time he had been paralyzed from his neck downward. I greeted him in his hospital room. He was much thinner than before. His once muscular arms were now wasted. He lay very still, explaining that any movement of his head caused severe pain and shocklike sensations in his extremities. He hurt all over. He was afraid that he might cough or sneeze again. He expressed his hope that we could help him.

Farmers have a unique approach to dealing with illnesses and injuries; they are both more realistic and more accepting. My father-in-law raised corn, soybeans, and Angus cattle on his southern Illinois farm, despite the loss of his dominant right arm in a shooting accident in early manhood. When he sustained a heart attack, neighboring farmers simply added his chores to their own, and he in turn reciprocated during times of their illnesses. If his increasingly arthritic left hand ached or if his muscles were stiff from hard work, he never complained. Long days in the sun gave him a perpetual mild squint as he leaned against a wooden gate and quietly pondered a planted field or promising bull. He remained quietly in charge of his life until his own death from myeloma.

Clyde and my father-in-law, experts in matters of nature, knew how to look directly into the face of illness. They'd say things like "Get to the point. Tell me straight up. I know about life and the seasons with all their unpredictability."

Each step in Clyde's evaluation brought the grimmest of results— his bones were riddled with malignant lesions; his bone marrow was replaced with sheets of bizarre plasma cells. Every therapy then available had been employed.

Bob Heyssel led the clinical team that month. He had earlier hunted quail with Clyde. Bob worked out of a typical junior faculty office, with its green boxes of investigative reprints whose quantity determined academic promotion. Bob and another hematologist, John Flexner, served as Clyde's personal physicians.

After reviewing with me Clyde's blood and marrow smears and his x-rays with their punched-out lesions of bone, Bob thought aloud about his patient and his overwhelming illness. No further chemotherapy or radiation was feasible. The two of us went to Clyde's bedside in a four-bed unit. I pulled the curtain around Clyde's space. The farmer and the academic hematologist shared a stripped down conversational style. They chatted for a few moments. I stood aside with the uneasiness of a house doctor who worries that his facial expression may prematurely give away bad news.

Clyde asked, "Is this it, Doc?"

"Yes, I think so," the hematologist said.

The hematology professor sat on the end of Clyde's bed, pulled out a cigarette from the pack in his shirt pocket, and lit up. After a puff or two he passed the cigarette to Clyde who smoked it the rest of the way.

It was time for Clyde to go home. He would require bed rest and would not be able to move very much. Nurses would travel to the farm each day to assist Clyde's wife in his care. His pain would be controlled. All of this would be discussed with Clyde's wife when she arrived at the hospital later that day.

There was silence as Clyde finished the cigarette. He spoke of shared quail hunts.

"You'll have to come up there sometime," he said as he looked at me. He shook both of our hands, taking care to avoid movement of his head and neck, then he thanked us. An ambulance took him home the following day.

Clyde's wife phoned a few days later to report his death.

Bob Heyssel and John Flexner attended the funeral in rural Tennessee. There was an open casket. Clyde's immediate and extended family waited their turn to kiss his forehead before the casket was sealed. Thirty years later Bob Heyssel remembered the scene vividly.

I learned many scientific facts during my two-month stint on the hematology service. I read and thought intensively about megakaryocytes and the maturational sequence of leukocytes and the metabolism of folic acid. Because the hematology service had a particular interest in paroxysmal nocturnal hemoglobinuria, I learned more than I would ever need to know about that disorder. The notes are around somewhere. I know where to look and whom to ask when I encounter a hematology question. But what I learned that day on that service had to do with style. This style is not a veneer or a glibness to be acquired by imitation or from the reading of a manual on public relations. It has to do rather with the persistent and unflinching awareness of a shared humanity, which finally dissolves all barriers when speaking and listening to one another.

FIREMAN DOCTOR

"My daddy is a fireman doctor."

Will Cleaveland achieved instant celebrity in the eyes of his fellow four-year-olds at Scarritt College's pre-kindergarten. The children had been asked, in turn, to describe their father's work. Will's teacher checked the accuracy of his boast with my wife. Will was correct—to a point.

After two Nashville fireman had sustained myocardial infarctions while fighting blazes, the city fathers and Vanderbilt clinical nutrition-ists collaborated on a project aimed at improving the health of the men of the fire halls. Three fire companies comprised the study group. In-vestigators measured baseline cholesterol and glucose levels, estimated body fat from determinations of skin-fold thickness, checked electro-cardiograms, and finally assessed performance of the men in various physical tasks. The initial phase was followed by weeks of supervised exercise from 6:00 to 7:00 A.M., five days per week. The chemical and physical assessments were repeated at intervals. The firemen received counseling in healthful diets and smoking cessation. A graduate student in exercise physiology supervised each morning's exercise session; a medical resident provided clinical oversight. Ever in need of additional income in those days of $200 per month paychecks, I signed up for

$10 per session.

Most of the firemen were out of shape. Many worked two jobs hoping for an interval of paid sleep while on duty at the fire station. Most of the men smoked. Several were quite obese. Their ages ranged from mid-20s to 60. At the initial exercise session I watched the men struggle and gasp to complete their aerobic workouts. I worried that we would precipitate more myocardial infarctions than we prevented. One particularly obese older fireman flushed and sweated profusely but ignored my entreaty that he sit down and rest for a while. There was the matter of pride; to stop or even slow down would cost a man in the eyes of his fellows. A few of the men comfortably completed the workout; the rest seemed near collapse at the one-hour mark. Hopefully, they would not be called to an emergency before their shift ended.

Repeated radio transmissions from a central fire dispatcher provided a background for the exercise. Sometimes, a loud, harsh buzz alerted the men that their ladder company was needed. Within less than a minute the fire engines roared from the hall while the crew pulled on their boots and heavy overalls. I sensed that the firemen welcomed the release from the grueling workouts. Trucks might return after a few minutes if the alarm had been false. At other times the crews were away for the remainder of the hour. They would describe each blaze to me the following morning in the most casual of tones.

The firemen and I enjoyed instant trust. Rather than medical onlooker, I became a de facto battalion surgeon. Skin lesions, colds, muscular aches, a swollen joint, and a hernia were brought to my attention.

"Hey, Doc, what have you got for..." and there followed a description of a cough or sinus congestion or problem with bladder or bowel. Most requests were voiced loudly. Occasionally, at the end of an exercise session, a fireman would take me aside and, in a whisper, describe a urethral discharge or some problem encountered in intercourse. Complaints from wives, children, and in-laws were relayed for my judgment and comment. From the outset of the program and with no hesitancy the men brought to me their complaints, even of the most intimate nature.

Had no one taken the health concerns of these men seriously before? Did they lack funds or insurance to permit medical evaluations? Or was it the long hours of work that precluded medical inquiry?

Shoulders and lower backs were the principal casualties of our exercise programs. As the workout progressed these complaints diminished and even the most rotund and out-of-shape firemen showed definite improvement in strength, agility, and speed. The camaraderie rivaled that of a team in a locker room.

When I described to Will a particular scene in which the fire trucks had roared from the hall to fight a large fire, I could see that I had assumed the stature of an astronaut in his eyes. In response to his request, we stopped by the fire hall one Saturday afternoon to look at the engines. We talked briefly with two of the firemen. Will was quiet, but his eyes said "Wow!" I stood at the pinnacle of pediatric esteem.

After a few months the project ended. Chemical and performance results were duly recorded, and the firemen and I returned to our prior pursuits. I doubt that we modified anyone's behavior. I suspect that, in light of the exhausting schedules, few of the firemen could afford the time and energy to continue any systematic program of exercise. From time to time, in a mall or in the hallways of the hospital, I briefly encountered a fireman from our group.

"Hey, Doc," was the standard greeting. I might be told a joke or asked for advice. I might be told about a particularly tough two- or three-alarm blaze. None of the men ever indicated apprehension or anxiety. This was simply their job.

When I was a boy, the LaGrange Fire Department acquired, at the end of World War II, a beautiful new American-La France truck with a mechanical extension ladder. The new machine was displayed on the square and, after the crowd of adults and children had circled the brilliant red vehicle, the steel ladder was extended to the top of the three-story bank building. Firemen scurried up the ladder to fight a mock blaze signaled by a yellow smoke pot atop the structure. I was dazzled.

Twenty years later, I was briefly a fireman doctor. Will Cleaveland and I considered this my niftiest job.

TOO TOUGH FOR ME

Once, the professor stood before grand rounds at the Veterans Administration Hospital to discuss a case of chronic lymphocytic leukemia. In two minutes he gave a capsule synopsis of the then-accepted protocol for chemotherapy for the disorder. He asked if there were any questions, and there being none he descended the podium and walked toward the exit. Just as he prepared to leave the auditorium, a fellow resident stood to protest. "Wait a minute, Dr. Brittingham, you don't really believe that. What's going on?"

The professor paused and, turning toward his audience, challenged us to pick apart the standard protocol. Rather than ascend the podium, he walked among his audience. During the next 45 minutes we thought corporately of chronic lymphocytic leukemia and its various complications. We felt secure accepting a strategy of careful, watchful waiting for asymptomatic patients. Premature chemotherapy shortened the lives of patients so afflicted.

The great teachers challenge us to reach deep inside to examine our assumptions. He was the greatest.

When a patient was to be presented at twice-weekly professor's rounds, he searched out old records, even if this meant traveling to nearby hospitals to read clinical charts. He questioned relatives closely and culled data from hometown physicians who had referred patients to Vanderbilt Hospital. Whether a clinical case was presented by a third-year medical student in a clerkship or a first-year resident, he never criticized or belittled the performance. The presenter was a colleague, and together they would establish a diagnosis and define a course of treatment. When a student or house officer established a useful point or found a new clue to the illness at hand, his standard response was, "You guys are too tough for me!"

As I accompanied him down a hallway one day, a student newly assigned to a medical rotation stopped us and hesitatingly asked a question relevant to a patient on his ward. "Let's find out," the professor stated. We detoured to the library where, over the next 30 minutes, the three of us covered a table with journals and textbooks and worked out an answer to the question.

In my final year of residency, a physician from a community in southern Kentucky phoned to solicit my help in arranging for his patient's admission to Dr. Brittingham's service. The referring physician described his patient as the wife of a prominent local business owner. She was totally disabled by headaches.

Ordinarily, the professor limited his personal practice to a handful of faculty members and their spouses. He agreed to accept a new patient this time.

I greeted the patient upon her arrival. She was the quintessential, plasticized trophy wife. A review of systems in her medical history was positive for every complaint. Subsequently, Dr. Brittingham spent two hours questioning and examining the troubled woman. I was surprised when he immediately discharged her from the hospital. He explained to her, "I'm sorry. I can't help you."

We adopted his means of inquiry; we did not want to disappoint our mentor's faith in us as physicians or physicians-to-be. His standards were high, and he called us to emulate them but always with smiles and gentle encouragement.

All of the many cases that he had examined over the years he catalogued in pencil on 3" × 5" index cards. From these he derived fresh insights into the immune deficiencies of patients who had lost their spleens. He early predicted the hepatic toxicity of isoniazid, which was used at that time in a cavalier fashion to treat patients with positive skin tests for tuberculosis.

A particularly severe migraine kept me from work one morning. I felt my head would explode. My wife consulted Dr. Brittingham, who asked that I be brought to his office. Following a thorough and gentle examination, he sought my wife's opinion about what was wrong with my health.

"I think he's working too hard."

He agreed with her diagnosis and advised me to take a couple of days off.

For three years I shared with Dr. Brittingham Monday afternoon duty in the medical clinic at Nashville General Hospital. We residents worked feverishly to see our 10 to 12 patients in the chronically overworked and understaffed clinic. The professor routinely saw 20 or more patients. When he was away one afternoon, we pinch-hit for him. From one patient I learned that the professor had purchased her eyeglasses, from another I learned of his payment for needed dental work.

After years of teaching, the professor changed the direction of his career. In a letter to me, he stated that he had become "a little tired" and wanted to see what full-time practice was all about. He joined a small medical group in Fort Worth. I wrote from time to time and received letters that reflected the same intense clinical inquiry, always tinted with good humor.

The physician who assumed responsibility for Dr. Brittingham's patients after his departure for Texas told me of other beneficences. Soon after he took charge of the professor's patients, the nurse in the clinic told the new physician that it was time to visit a homebound patient. Dr. Brittingham called upon the homebound lady each month, delivering to her a supply of medications drawn from the clinic's closet of samples. The new doctor gathered the medical supplies and drove to a nearby housing project. A frail aged lady greeted him. She expressed her gratitude as he handed over the medications.

"But where are my groceries?" she asked.

Years into my Chattanooga practice a friend from Nashville telephoned. The professor had renal cell carcinoma that had metastasized widely. The friend had no further details.

I called his office in Texas—it would be 9:00 A.M. there—in hopes of learning more from one of the professor's medical partners. Instead, the office receptionist connected me immediately to my teacher. This was his final day in the office.

"You know, Clifton, I needed a good third-year medical student, someone like David Dodson (my friend and partner, whom he highly regarded). I had a pain in my hip for three years, and I thought it was arthritic. It was the darndest thing. I had a CT scan, and the tumor is already in my liver and my bones."

I didn't know what to say. I expressed sympathy, I think.

"I'm not afraid of checking out. Not a bit. I just needed one of you guys to tell me what was wrong." We talked for a few more moments about shared experiences on the medical service at Vanderbilt and what different colleagues were up to in their careers. We reviewed the activities of our children.

"I can never thank you guys enough," he said. And we bade our good-byes.

A few months later he died at home.

The headstone in the family cemetery reads:

BELOVED PHYSICIAN
THOMAS EVANS BRITTINGHAM
February 2, 1924
July 27, 1986
In my end is my beginning.

His picture is on the wall of my office, signed "With appreciation," as he signed every picture given to the house officers—his colleagues and friends—who requested one. Teaching as exemplified by Tom Brittingham, the professor, is an act of love. It is also an act of deep appreciation for the privilege of the search and the company of the curious, the motivated, and the compassionate.

FORT KNOX

1968-1970

AMERICA has maintained its own iron curtains at various times, and I slipped behind one in July 1968. Barring severe physical impairment, all physicians could expect a two-year tour of duty in either the armed forces or the public health service. After the anxiety of the Match for internship positions, we faced a second, randomized lottery that would assign the branch and time of entry into uniformed service. This was the Berry Plan, which determined whether induction would occur after internship or after completion of a residency. Presumably, the latter selection would ensure the opportunity of practice in one's specialty. In 1964 I received a four-year deferment for service in the Medical Corps of the U.S. Army.

The national mood toward the Vietnam War was souring progressively by early 1968. In January the Vietcong had unleashed a devastating offensive, which coincided with the Tet celebration of the lunar new year. Anti-war sentiment on campuses, already seething with rage, intensified, and demonstrations broke out even at placid southern universities such as Vanderbilt. A young female neighbor had been cited for breaking the arm of a campus policeman during such a protest. One Sunday night we listened with amazement as Lyndon

Johnson announced his withdrawal from further campaigning for re-election. Our embattled national administration seemed incapable of action as the times became more ominous and unsettling.

By April I had yet to learn about my forthcoming military assignment and I could make no plans. Phone calls on my behalf by my chairman led to the recommendation that I travel to Washington for interviews that might lead to a favorable assignment. I flew into National Airport two mornings after the assassination of Martin Luther King Jr. No taxis waited outside the airport, and I had to walk into the city. The wail of sirens, both distant and near, and plumes of smoke from distant buildings testified to the chaos of anguished protests. Once in the city I repeatedly phoned the offices where my interviews were to occur. No one seemed to know anything about them; the Army colonel I was to meet was unavailable. I returned home the following day.

Days before my residency ended, I was instructed to report to Fort Knox in 30 days. Because of a shortage of physicians, my basic training would be deferred.

Our sons—Rance, Will, Mark, and Tom—believed they had been transported to a perpetual theme park. Besides having a wonderful creek with crawdads at the foot of their backyard, they could play in the ancient and new tanks in the base's museum and watch helicopters aloft and parades on the ground. They could stand at attention at 5:00 P.M., when the gun atop a tank fired, bugles sounded, and colors were lowered at the parade ground.

Fort Knox's population swelled to 75,000, basic trainees and students in the elementary and advanced armor courses. Ironically, General Heinz Guderian, who had led Hitler's Panzer divisions against the United States in World War II, served as a visiting lecturer to the young armor students. At night the horizon rumbled and flared from the rounds fired during perpetual maneuvers. Once, I sat in a large grandstand with congressmen and civilian and military dignitaries to watch a simulated attack by Sheridan tanks, Huey attack helicopters, and missile-firing jets tearing the air above us. This was the embodiment of the armed conflict dramatized by every war movie I had ever watched.

Away from the action sentiments were deeply contorted. Young men who had been drafted brought dread and anti-war sentiments as part of their emotional baggage. I knew of young men who donned long-haired wigs so that they would not be identified as soldiers when they used 48-hour passes in nearby Louisville. Cafes and coffee houses beyond the perimeter of the reservation were alleged to be centers of anti-war activity, and we were told that the Army monitored who came and went. The Army tried to seal us hermetically from the nation's swirling political tides.

As physicians our lot was somewhat different. Clinics for dependents and military retirees, though packed, functioned well because of the assigned corpsmen and nurses. Ireland Army Hospital provided care for the sick and injured among the active duty personnel and their wives and children. Most nights, an air evacuation plane brought casualties from Vietnam for further care. The large hospital could provide a level of care similar to that of the hospitals in which we had trained.

We remained woefully understaffed on the medical service. Half of us had entered military service following deferments under the Berry Plan, which permitted the completion of our medical training; the other half had been drafted after years in civilian practice. Our departmental commander was the lone career military internist, and he stayed out of our way. We became the professional equivalent of a pick-up team that, despite random and haphazard selection of its members, nonetheless seeks to perform in a proud way. Indeed, we formed our own faculty of medicine complete with journal clubs, morning reports, and grand rounds. Within our clique we felt somewhat aloof from the formal and sometimes preposterous pressures emanating from the military establishment. We used the term "doctor" rather than the "captain" or "major" of our ranks. There were still limits which, if we stepped beyond, we knew would trigger our immediate posting to Vietnam. A young colleague who was abruptly transferred to Vietnam suspected that this was punishment for remarks critical of the military that his wife had made in a letter mailed to a foreign friend. Clearly, we lived within a small police state in which we were to work hard, perform our military duties, and keep a low profile.

In May 1970 I spent a weekend of leave at the annual show-and-tell meetings of America's medical research establishment in Atlantic City. A lunch was interrupted by news of the fatal shooting by National Guardsmen of four students during an anti-war protest at Kent State. The fabric of a civil society seemed to be unraveling continually. The civilian and military components of our nation were dangerously out of touch with one another, and for a while the military would continue to function in a way that seemed freed of Constitutional reins.

In July 1970 my two-year obligation for military service was completed. From a medical standpoint, I had seen and learned amazing things: multiple cases of malaria and exotic parasitic infections from Southeast Asia, dozens of cases of meningococcal meningitis, complicated infections of wounds infected by feces-coated booby traps. I had worked with doctors who sustained lofty professional standards within an intolerant environment. I had been fortunate to remain with my family in the states throughout. But more clearly than ever before I saw that, as physicians, we cannot practice within an ethical or political vacuum. We are obligated to participate as citizens in each of the multiple layers of community in which we live. The duty to work toward a just and moral society is no less than our obligation to learn and to practice excellent medicine.

THE GREAT POISON
IVY CAPER

Too many John Wayne movies had distorted my expectations for military service. The beginning of my two-year military obligation was hardly auspicious. A rotund colonel with a fixed look of disdain hardly acknowledged my presence as he handed over my duty assignments. I would begin each day at the stockade dispensary. After an hour, I would report to the WAC dispensary and then proceed to the medical clinic for dependents. After lunch I would alternate afternoons in the emergency room with duty on the inpatient service. Because of a shortage of physicians, basic training was postponed indefinitely. Something was said about maintaining a positive attitude. I was in the Army now, and I should never forget that fact. I should obtain my uniforms that afternoon and report to work the following morning. The colonel returned his gaze to the papers atop his desk. I assumed that was my cue for dismissal.

"And don't be late," he warned as I left his office.

By imitation I learned when I should salute and where to pin the various insignia. Corpsmen and nurses, sensing my unease, proffered additional advice. I felt as if I were starting work in a discount department store rather than the U.S. Army.

Quickly, the days fell into a routine not unlike housestaff time. I even had duty every fourth night in the emergency room. I was promised compensation time sometime in the far, misty future. Patients streamed in at each locale, and no one in authority took much notice of my presence or bothered me.

A few days later I was summoned to the dyspeptic colonel's office. In addition to my present chores, I would henceforth serve as the physician member of a team that would investigate crashes of any military aircraft in the region. He handed me a manual which would explain my duties.

"Don't worry. We don't have any crashes."

And then came my first "special assignment."

The rising senior class from West Point arrived, as they did each summer, to visit our base, ostensibly to learn firsthand the functions in combat of tanks and the many other forms of armor, the specialty of Fort Knox. This also was a prime opportunity, a rush party really, to interest the future leaders of America's Army in careers in this branch of service. Cadets received full celebrity treatment from the post's senior brass. Intense days in the field during their short visit would be followed on their final evening by a formal dinner and dance. Young women imported from Louisville and surrounding communities would join the eligible daughters of officers at this glittering military cotillion.

No one anticipated the effects of poison ivy.

Southerners learn early to avoid poison ivy. "Keep out of the road. Don't play with matches. And watch out for the poison ivy." The compound leaf of *Rhus radicans* may be accompanied by small white berries early in the spring before the leaves turn crimson in the fall. Once, a visitor from New York to my Georgia home gathered the lovely red, autumnal leaves of the toxic weed to press into the pages of a book, only to break out in a severe rash the following day.

Northern Kentucky's summer had been unusually wet, encouraging luxuriant growth of poison ivy everywhere: fences, ground wires, open and wooded spaces were covered with the green carpet. Apparently, the young cadets were bivouacked in the middle of the mother of all poison ivy patches. Perhaps the cadets were unfamiliar with the weed or in the dark did not realize their contact with it. In any event, in mid-afternoon preceding the gala, the emergency unfolded.

Again I was summoned to the grumpy colonel's office. I was being pulled from the emergency room to deal with a crisis involving the West Point cadets. Two corpsmen and I would leave immediately to open a special dispensary. A pharmacist with a chest of medicines would accompany us. I was advised to be respectful; these were special patients. The exact nature of the crisis remained obscure, something about a skin allergy. My first special assignment in the military was under way. Move over, John Wayne.

Within minutes, the ever efficient corpsman had activated the dispensary, and a few minutes later the first cadets arrived by bus. More than a hundred eventually came.

Never have I seen such severe poison ivy dermatitis affecting so many people at one time. There were blisters and bullae, rashes on hands and necks, shoulders and trunks. Some cadets appeared to have rolled naked on the botanical carpet. Several had swollen faces and reddened eyes. Had they been downwind of burning ivy? Despite obvious discomfort from the itchy rash, the young men maintained the proud posture and clipped answers of West Point cadets. Ironically, after managing for three years the rigorous academic, cultural, and physical demands of officer training, they had been defeated by a poisonous weed. They had encountered a new form of biological warfare, and this on their native soil.

The cadets lined up in various stages of undress before my table. The sign at the dispensary entrance stated, "Before you can see the doctor, the affected part must be exposed," and the cadets were not about to violate any regulation. I examined each briefly. We doled out steroid creams for the milder cases, gave injections to the more severely affected, and dispatched two of the young soldiers to the hospital for intravenous steroid therapy.

After an hour, the sole dermatologist on the medical staff, a career officer, put in a cameo appearance.

"Goddammit, Captain," he addressed me. "You're taking too much time. Give everybody a shot and get them out of here. They're having dinner with the General."

Thus ordered, the corpsman and I cranked up a therapeutic assembly line and dispensed with the niceties of examining and talking to each patient.

Many seats of honor remained vacant at the night's social extravaganza at the Officer's Club. The urge to scratch probably dampened pleasures of the evening for many and may even have blighted nascent romances. I never learned how many cadets were lured to careers in armor that year. Given the penchant for the Army of that day to overreact to adversity, I was surprised that napalm-laden aircraft were not called in to rid the base of the pesky weed. I leave to some future archivist the formal correlations between career choice and intensity of itch.

CURING INFERTILITY

My only documented success in curing infertility occurred at Fort Knox. That morning in the medical clinic for dependents was quite typical. Every chair in the waiting area was filled with wives and older children mingled with military retirees from nearby communities. At best we could offer a quick look, the elicitation of a single complaint, and a brief examination of the affected body part before formulating a plan of action. We had time only to shoot from the holster and not from the hip.

The young woman appeared to be no more than 18. She was tall and slender and seemed quite anxious. Her bright red lipstick matched the broad ribbon that brought some order to her tightly curled blonde hair.

It was her turn to be seen.

"We can't have children." She choked back tears, while I thought of a quick referral to the Ob-Gyn Clinic.

She was 19, and she had been married to her second lieutenant husband for eight months and was not yet pregnant. She urgently wanted a child before her husband received the inevitable orders for Vietnam. He was in armor training. She knew that his next assignment would be perilous and that in a few weeks they would begin an extended interval apart. Throughout the brief visit in the examination cubicle she dabbed at tears while her cheeks flushed intensely. Her soft voice repeatedly cracked.

Referral to the gynecologist would require some days, and she did not wish to wait. She implored me to do something, to outline a course of action. She would be willing to see a civilian gynecologist if necessary, although she worried about the expense this might entail.

The clinic nurse helped her into an examination gown while I saw other patients. As I re-entered her cubicle, I sought other information. Onset of puberty and menstrual cycles had been entirely normal. She denied ever using birth control pills. Her husband's health was vigorous.

"And how often do you have intercourse?"

My nurse could not totally conceal her gasp as the reply came, "Three times a day." I stopped scribbling my clinical notes.

"And how long have you maintained this pattern of three time a day intercourse?"

"Since we were married."

In a clinic of such volume and diversity of patients, I was accustomed to surprise. An immobile countenance was a prerequisite for a physician in that clinic. This was indeed a new dimension to the procreative urge, which had pushed us forward through the millennia.

I did not need to examine her. After she had dressed we spoke briefly. I suggested that she limit intercourse, at least for a month, to no more than three times per week. I pulled that number from the air. She was downcast, worrying that her husband would not understand this strategy of rationing. But I persisted. "Three times a week, and I think you will have a good chance to become pregnant."

Later that day I was called urgently to the telephone in the emergency room where I was assigned for the afternoon. The clerk whispered a warning that the caller was quite upset.

"Captain, you are trying to hurt my marriage." It was the hypercopulative second lieutenant. His voice trembled with anger. Neither he nor his marriage could endure such restrictions. I heard him out. He shared his wife's desire for children, and, yes, a pregnancy before his shipping out to Vietnam would be wonderful. I argued that since an appointment with the obstetrician-gynecologist would require time, why not try my strategy? He wanted to know the source of my recommendation. I replied that my advice was derived from my own rotation in obstetrics during medical school. And I did have such a vague recollection. He was not to be placated.

In the rush of patients and events over the next several weeks, I had occasional chuckles whenever I recalled this scenario. My thoughts shifted to other patients.

Several weeks later another phone call came to my clinic. It was the teenage bride, and she was pregnant. She had had no further menstrual periods after the clinic visit. Rationing of lovemaking, though difficult and not entirely adhered to, had worked nonetheless. She was queasy at the time of her first missed period, and soon afterward sensed that a fetus was present. Her husband had received orders for an assignment in Vietnam.

"I feel wonderful." She would move soon to her hometown to wait out her husband's tour of foreign duty.

The experience in that busy place, in that time of war and social upheaval, could be compared to standing on a busy train platform on a holiday weekend with swirls of people moving in all directions at great speed. Occasionally, in such a setting, a face or figure stands out in the crowd but in a moment is gone. The enlisted men and young officers received orders for Vietnam. Their wives and children returned to civilian homes to wait and to worry.

The second lieutenant remained but a voice over the telephone, irritated that his prolonged honeymoon was no more. The odds are strong that he survived a rotation of duty to Southeast Asia. His body would have had the additional protection of thick armor plate. His wife I saw but once. Pretty and anxious, she could have served nobly as cheerleader for any high school or college. But this ritual of postadolescence was not to be. War prompted hurried courtships and truncated dreams.

I hope the infant was healthy and joined later by brothers and sisters, with the father back home in some Midwestern community to love and care for their mother and them.

ELEANOR

⁂

She was brought by her mother to the morning medical clinic at the Fort Knox Hospital where I had worked for only a few weeks. She was 16, too old for the pediatric clinic, and she complained of being fatigued all of the time. Her mother noted that her daughter seemed pale and as if she had lost a few pounds from her already slender frame.

Because of an ongoing deluge of patients we had scant minutes for the retirees and families of active duty personnel at our base. Our clinic served the functions of both triage and definitive care. Sometimes, two physicians would see 100 or more patients in the morning hours allotted to civilians. While one of us screened patients and tended to minor complaints, the other would address more complex problems. Against a background of such frantic motion, the last thing I needed was a patient with vague complaints. Give me a cellulitis or a thyroid nodule or a congested lung.

I listened to Eleanor's story. She lived on the military reservation with her mother and officer-father. She felt constantly tired and dreaded getting out of bed each morning. She could not concentrate and feared that she would do poorly in class once her 11th grade classes began. She demanded good grades of herself. Although this was summer vacation, she had no desire to go swimming or to participate in any outdoor activities. There was no fever, cough, nausea, or diarrhea. Her last menstrual period had occurred months earlier.

Her eyes demanded contact throughout my examination. She was friendly, though reserved, and answered my questions politely. She weighed barely 100 pounds. Apart from evidence of weight loss and pallor, I found nothing else on my physical examination, no enlargement of lymph nodes or spleen. Did I note an element of fear in her hazel eyes?

I ordered a blood count, a test for infectious mononucleosis, and an assay of hepatic enzymes. At the conclusion of the few minutes allotted for this examination, I told Eleanor and her mother that I would be in touch as soon as I had some answers.

Before the floodgates opened to patients the next morning, I reviewed the previous day's lab work. Eleanor's blood counts were abnormal. Her white count was elevated to the mid-20,000 range; the majority of these white cells were described as very atypical lymphocytes. Later that day I took the slide and the report to a hematologist assigned to a nearby research unit. After review of the slide he, too, commented on the unusual features of the average-sized but highly atypical white cells.

"Get a marrow," he recommended.

I explained the situation to Eleanor's mother, who accompanied her daughter to the clinic the next morning. They wished to proceed with the test. Eleanor was slender enough that a marrow from the iliac crest was no problem. She was unafraid and seemed to have little discomfort during the procedure. Good technique? Or a patient determined to show little emotion?

Our pathologist was puzzled by the microscopic appearance of Eleanor's bone marrow. The research hematologist was not. He stated, "Micromyeloblasts. Send her to Walter Reed."

Sometimes things are not as they seem, and I had that feeling now. Apart from appearing wan, Eleanor looked every bit the typical young woman in her mid-teens. She was not anemic, nor were her platelets reduced. Perhaps she had acute leukemia in a pre-symptomatic phase. Certainly, she did not resemble any leukemic patient whom I had encountered during my residency years at Vanderbilt. The microscopic appearance of her peripheral blood and bone marrow did not quite fit with those in the hematology atlas that I consulted. My teachers during residency had repeatedly urged a course of watchful waiting when clinical studies seemed contradictory or nonsensical. This was clearly such a time.

I summoned Eleanor and her mother to the clinic. This time, for whatever reason, Eleanor wanted her mother to remain in the lobby, while the nurse and I examined her. Eleanor, as always, was polite and reserved but soon tears filled her eyes and spilled down her cheeks.

"Do you want us to get your mother?" I asked.

"No," she replied. "Can the nurse leave?"

I nodded, and the nurse somewhat reluctantly stepped outside the curtained examination cubicle.

"I vomit. I make myself vomit," Eleanor said.

For months Eleanor, after completing breakfast, had gone to the bathroom to induce vomiting by sticking her forefinger down her throat. She had begun the practice before school had adjourned for the summer. After lunch she vomited again, and she did it yet again after raiding the refrigerator for snacks following her return home in mid-afternoon. Sometimes she sneaked into the kitchen in the middle of the night to eat before repeating the sequence in her upstairs bathroom. Her waking hours were filled with dread that her compulsion would be discovered.

"Don't tell my mother," she pleaded.

"We must," I said.

We were at a standoff. A frail, early structure of rapport was in danger of collapse. We negotiated a truce: I would not tell her mother just yet in exchange for her best efforts to stop the vomiting. Both ends of the deal held. She balked, however, at my recommendation that she must seek psychiatric counsel.

Could the repeated vomiting cause the abnormality in her blood and bone marrow? There was little clinical information then regarding bulimia, which subsequently was to develop celebrity status among illnesses. The hematologist said there was no known association and that I should simply ship the patient to Louisville or to Walter Reed Army Hospital.

I waited. Perhaps repeated vomiting had caused vitamin deficiency. I called her mother and suggested the addition of a daily multivitamin.

A week later Eleanor, to my wishful eye, appeared less tired and pale. Her blood count was improved; the white count had fallen, and the percentage of abnormal cells had decreased as well.

"What have you done with the girl with leukemia?" The call came from the research hematologist.

"I'm watching her." I explained my follow-up observations.

"You know she's a major's daughter?" he asked.

"Yes."

A week later Eleanor's blood counts had improved still further, and over the subsequent weeks of that long-ago summer her blood picture returned to normal.

Our understaffed base had but one psychiatrist, and mental health services were severely strained. Psychological counsel could be arranged sometimes for military dependents in civilian offices outside the military reservation. Eleanor remained uninterested in any type of formal counseling. She continued to insist that neither her mother nor her father were to know the nature of her illness. She assured me that she no longer vomited. I urged her to take the next step, and ask herself why she felt such a powerful need to throw up. By this time her junior year of high school had begun. She was happier, and she reported that her academic work thrived. Her life seemed on track for a banner academic year.

In mid-winter Eleanor appeared with abdominal pain and had typical appendicitis. She recovered quickly from surgery.

At her bedside, I asked the physician's generic question as to how things were going.

She no longer vomited. She felt that she would soon have to run away, however.

"You must let me speak with your parents."

"They wouldn't understand. They would never forgive me."

I insisted upon a meeting with the family. She wanted only her mother present. At the meeting, held before Eleanor's discharge from the hospital, I indicated that Eleanor had acknowledged overwhelming stress, and I advised psychological evaluation. Eleanor left the hospital.

Later her mother indicated that Eleanor seemed happier, but the young woman steadfastly refused to meet with any counselor.

In the tumult of too many patients and too few doctors, I could think of Eleanor occasionally but only briefly before some new set of demands took my time.

Early one spring morning I sat in the tiny office assigned to me along with additional responsibilities. My secretary came in, her usual calmness disturbed by something.

"There is a young girl to see you. Something's the matter with her."

She ushered Eleanor into my office. A facial towel was wrapped about one wrist. There was dried blood on the other sleeve of her blouse. I assured my secretary that everything was under control, and I invited Eleanor to sit down and talk.

She sobbed. She felt unworthy of the love of anyone, family or friends alike.

"You mustn't tell."

Religious worship meant much to Eleanor and her family. She loved the music of the church and its formalized traditions. She had learned to play the flute as a child, adding her musical zest to worship services. At 12 or thereabouts a teacher, a middle-aged woman of the church, befriended her and took extra delight in Eleanor's musical precocity. Eleanor was invited to remain alone with the teacher after group activities adjourned. They might sing or watch television. The teacher placed her arm around Eleanor one afternoon and pulled her close to kiss her deeply on her lips. Subsequent meetings led to further kisses and intimate caresses. Eleanor sensed the danger, and she felt that her actions were awful but longed for the intimacy. Her waking hours were dominated by thoughts of when she would next meet her teacher.

"You must never tell." This had been the final admonition from her lover just before Eleanor's family was transferred to Fort Knox.

I examined her wrist. Her wounds were not serious, a series of deep scratches had been drawn by the paring knife. I cleaned and dressed her wounds. She agreed to psychiatric counsel.

Subsequently, I received several letters from Eleanor as she received inpatient care in a civilian psychiatric clinic. Even in the depths of sadness, Eleanor had a muted sense of joy just waiting to happen. The letters spoke of music, of new friends, and of 19th century European novels she was reading. She especially relished Dostoevsky.

A year later I completed my military stint and left for Nashville and a clinical fellowship. A further letter from Eleanor spoke of her return to her senior year in a high school adjacent to the military base. Her father had been posted to Vietnam. I kept her address and six months later I called Eleanor's residence during a trip to Louisville. Eleanor answered and invited me to stop by. I had never seen her fully happy before. Her eyes sparkled. She was animated. She was no longer thin. She spoke of classes and books and plans for college.

Years later, I received a note from Eleanor. "My life is complete now." A year or so later another note arrived, this one from her mother telling me of Eleanor's death in an accident.

What happened in my work with Eleanor is what often happens with patients. That which is apparent, an abnormal blood smear in Eleanor's case, has nothing at all to do with what is truly wrong. Perhaps modern day technology can establish a clear link between abnormal white cells that mimicked leukemia and the young woman whose sorrow repeatedly drove her to thrust her finger down her throat to remove a previous meal. My vitamin pills were a stab into a dark mystery, and they possibly contributed to a restored, healthy bone marrow. I do not know. Misdirected passion from a church teacher, who must have suffered enormous terrors and stresses herself, was the first domino to fall. A vulnerable young girl was the next. I will never know to what level of happiness Eleanor could have reached. The spectrum of options for handling emotional chaos is so very limited for children in their teen years. For some reason, as I think of Eleanor the metaphor of swimming to shore through choppy seas springs to my mind. I see this young woman, exhausted, staggering onto the beach, and raising her arms in triumph.

OF RAZOR BLADES
AND LICE

The dispensary at the stockade was otherworldly. Most of the inmates had either gotten into fights or drunk too much alcohol in their hours off duty. Some other detainees, overwhelmed by thoughts of home and girlfriends, had gone AWOL, only to be returned to an environment far harsher than the barracks of basic training. An occasional addict had been arrested by military police as he used his stash of illicit drugs that he had smuggled onto the base.

One recruit from Detroit told me how he had been brought before a judge in criminal court on drug charges and been given the choice between imprisonment and enlistment in the military. He had been hospitalized because of bizarre behavior while on basic training maneuvers. While in the hospital he became wildly euphoric. A search by MPs of his belongings uncovered a cache of heroin hidden in the battery compartment of his portable radio.

Dispensary hours at the stockade began at 0700. My first duty was inspection of the half dozen prisoners held in solitary confinement. These men were the hardest-core offenders. They were kept in steel-meshed cages, sleeping upon wire springs on a concrete floor in the center of a large, central room. Their stark diets consisted of dry cereal, lettuce, some milk, meat, and potatoes. I was supposed to determine if they were malnourished or in any way unhealthy—this in a one- to two-minute visit.

Assaults against other prisoners and stockade guards constituted one main reason for solitary confinement. A couple of the inmates immediately waged war on their captors upon each release from their cages so that their time in captivity was spent in solitary confinement.

One prisoner was an exception. He had thrown a grenade into his lieutenant's tent while in Vietnam. I was not allowed into his cage. My daily inquiries as to his well-being elicited the foulest of verbal abuse. Later, because of especially violent behavior, he was transferred to a lock-up room at the hospital where he raged and stormed, throwing plates and trays at all who might enter, until he could be tied to his bed. One day he was transferred elsewhere.

The corpsman at the stockade dispensary battled alcoholism. This assignment was the last possible stop as he sought to qualify for his retirement pension before alcohol overwhelmed him. On most early mornings Listerine could not conceal the whiskey on his breath. I worried that any potentially addictive medications in the dispensary could not be trusted to him. Yet, if I blew the whistle on his misconduct, he would be court-martialed, and his career would be over. On two occasions at night while drunk he called my family's quarters, crying and telling me how his Vietnam tours had destroyed him. Once, I saw him quite inebriated as a patient in the hospital's emergency room. In the private little world, defined by the curtain pulled around his stretcher, he railed at the military, cursed the Vietcong, and spoke of atrocities that he had seen. I do not know if his reports were true.

He stated that once, while aboard a Huey helicopter with several soldiers and three blindfolded and bound Vietcong prisoners, he saw soldiers hurl two of the prisoners from the craft. The third was spared because he agreed to talk.

Finally, the corpsman and I reached an understanding. If he showed any evidence of alcohol use during my hour at the stockade, I would report him immediately. We would inventory controlled substances in the dispensary each morning, and if anything was missing, I would likewise turn him in. He would locate and attend Alcoholics Anonymous meetings each evening.

Because hospital time counted toward time served, the prisoners sought every way possible to gain admission to the hospital. Abdominal pain, chest pain, severe headache, shortness of breath—the challenge was to tease the few instances of true disease from the malingerings. Some prisoners would allege beatings from guards and sexual abuse from other prisoners. One day, three prisoners reported they had swallowed double-edged razor blades imbedded in pieces of bread. I sent them to the hospital emergency room where x-rays confirmed their claims. They were taken to surgery. The following day, additional blade swallowers were sent to the hospital. On the third day, those in command elected to withhold surgery and watch the next two metal ingesters. Surprisingly, the blades, which had been partially bent at the time of swallowing, passed in the stool without complication. Thus ended the brief Gillette epidemic.

One morning, at the end of my hour in the dispensary, I walked into the prison yard and confronted a guard as he kicked a prisoner in the flank while his charge performed push-ups. The guard glowered at me. I reported the incident immediately to the stockade commander, who promised that he would investigate. He also advised me that I should stick to doctoring and not meddle in the business of the prison.

The corpsman struggled meantime with the pressure of abstinence from alcohol. He became increasingly agitated and irritable. One morning, a new corpsman appeared. He reported that his predecessor had been transferred.

Another morning several of the prisoners at sick call complained of an itchy rash. I found lice on two of them. I reported my findings to the stockade commander who was furious and upbraided me as if I had imported the parasites to his facility. I learned immediately that, if there is one thing more feared by the military than poison gas, it is the body louse. In an administrative frenzy, uniforms, linens and mattresses—all things made of fabric—were gathered and burned. That was my last day of stockade duty at Fort Knox, Kentucky.

TOM'S KIDNEYS

Fear and sadness simultaneously hit me as the milky cloud of precipitant developed in the vial of fluid. I had added sulfosalicylic acid to a sample of urine from our 18-month-old son, Tom. I closed my eyes tightly and leaned against the counter in the lab before calling for help.

In the color photograph taken of our family that Saturday afternoon in our Fort Knox apartment, Ruzha and I are seated, flanked by Rance and Will. She holds three-year-old Mark in her lap, while an obviously edematous Tom sits in mine. The family photograph was a present from a retired sergeant whom I had treated for congestive heart failure.

Exactly how long Tom had been swollen is unclear. He had seemed fussy and tired for several days, but his appetite had remained voracious. He had had no fever. Earlier routine examinations had affirmed good health. As the photographer placed us for this portrait, I was aware that his face and feet were puffy. I suspect changes in his appearance had been underway for some time and were simply too subtle for us to notice.

As soon as the sitting ended we managed to capture from Tom a sample of urine, which I took immediately to the lab in the medical clinic. The lab was deserted. I dipped a chemical strip into the urine;

the protein reaction was strongly positive. I reached for the bottle of sulfosalicylic acid to confirm the finding. My hand was unsteady and I began to sweat. The solution became immediately opaque as I poured in the reagent. Tom had nephrosis.

Shaken, I returned home to explain to Ruzha that Tom was ill and likely would need hospitalization. I contacted the pediatrician on call for the hospital. After examining Tom, he recommended immediate admission.

Subsequent studies on our son, who rapidly became anuric, confirmed a severe nephrotic syndrome, attributable most likely to minimal change glomerulonephritis.

Did we wish Tom transferred elsewhere?

Pediatricians are cast from a different mold. In every setting, whether academic medical center or community hospital, civilian or military location, they exhibit the same expert love of children and the ability to calm and reassure both their young charges and their parents. The pediatricians of Fort Knox were no different. We elected to keep Tom under their care.

High-dose corticosteroids and bed rest comprised the treatment strategy. Initially, Tom occupied a crib with tall steel bars on the pediatric ward. Ruzha sat with him, reading and rocking him throughout the day. I joined them at lunch and after my work day concluded.

I, the father, prayed for his recovery. I, the physician, was skeptical of his chances and feared that Tom's renal disease would progress to death or a life-long need for high-dose steroid therapy. For the very first time, I faced serious illness within my own family. I wanted the miracle of a cure.

Tom improved and, after a week, returned home on a regimen of very limited activity. *Sesame Street* and added hours of being read to prompted his precocity in reading. Ruzha and I learned by heart the alphabet books from the Fort Knox Library. Frequent and careful monitoring by his pediatrician documented progressive improvement, although he would need steroids for a further six months. Mild relapses during the following two years required short-term courses of steroids. Apart from an episode of appendicitis, Tom's subsequent health has been uneventful.

Then, and at times of subsequent illnesses of our children, I experience almost unbearable conflict. Along with my wife, I need the informed comforting by an empathetic physician. I need the reassurance
that all that is reasonable is being done. At the same time the scientist
within me seeks insights into the disease process, and that invariably
means becoming aware of the worst possible outcomes. Reassurance
and fear compete. When one of my family members coughs or runs a
fever, my senses sharpen. Am I over-responding, or am I at risk of ig-
noring something potentially dangerous? Our clinical work keeps us
suspicious, observant, and uneasy, making it all but impossible to
maintain balanced judgment when the patient is one of our flesh and
blood.

The pediatrician's response to that 1969 phone call was prompt.
His examination was thorough. He subsequently sought fresh information from colleagues and a careful search of the literature. He addressed
us as parents, not as medical insiders. He anticipated our fears and tendered realistic expectations of therapy.

I could let go and move with my wife to the proper place for
parents in the presence of a sick child.

A SHATTERED DENTURE

ᐧᐧᐧ

In a curious turn of events, I worked for two weeks during the spring of 1970 in a United Mine Workers' hospital on the Kentucky-West Virginia border. The chronically understaffed facility actively recruited military physicians to spend off-duty days in its employment. Military leave time could be used in any fashion, and I needed the extra income of a locum tenens to apply to medical school loans. I needed a change of scenery as well from the rigidity of Fort Knox.

As I drove eastward into the coal fields the signs of poverty increased. The communities along the route seemed mired in a perpetual economic depression. My destination—Williamson, West Virginia—appeared faded and in need of paint and repair. I had entered a mining colony separated from much of the culture and prosperity of my nation. A new French restaurant presented a striking anomaly in the middle of the rundown town. Because of this area's early political support for John, and later Robert, Kennedy, the Kennedy Foundation had established the eatery as a training ground for young people in the area. Thus trained as waiters and chefs, the natives could seek well-paying jobs in prosperous cities in the Eastern United States. I do not know if the well-intended venture succeeded. Physicians at the hospital treated me to dinner at the restaurant one evening. We were the only diners and ordered from a menu whose prices were unaffordable for the great majority of the town's residents. The pleasant waitress, dressed as Hollywood might imagine a French girl on a festival day, had severely carious teeth. The experience was surreal and sad.

I checked into my quarters at the hospital on a Sunday evening and began work the next morning. The squat, dark structure had been flooded a few years earlier. The high-water mark on the walls was pointed out to me. Medical charts frequently bore the stamp "Old Records Lost in Flood." At meal time ambulatory patients helped in the service of food of barely palatable quality. The hospital belonged in a Third-World setting.

The medical clinic was filled with patients at 8:00 on my first morning. The nurse directed me to an acutely ill, groaning lady already wheeled into a treatment room. She writhed from side to side on the table. I could not estimate her age. Fifty? Or a worn and battered 30? She was malnourished and, like so many of the patients, had no teeth. A day earlier she had found at the roadside a dead possum, which she assumed had just been killed. She had dressed and cooked the animal and dined on its meat at supper. She had vomited repeatedly and had severe cramping throughout the night. At first light she struggled to reach the road where a neighbor gave her a ride to the clinic. I had no idea what illness I was treating. Fortunately, with intravenous fluids, antiemetics, and broad-spectrum antibiotics the lady improved. She left the hospital four days later, but to what?

I saw, in that gray place, gray and passive people who seemed exhausted. The older men had emphysema and deep bone rattling coughs. When they stood, they bent forward because of severe arthritis affecting necks, spines, and knees. Their faces were florid. Many suffered from diabetes and alcoholism.

The women appeared wasted, their countenances without expression. I sensed lives of sadness. There was whispered conversation in the waiting room. Individual patients volunteered little information. Throughout my days in the coal miners' hospital and clinic I was struck by the appalling lack of any medical knowledge among patients. Equally striking was the courtesy and gratitude expressed by each patient for even the most routine of care and advice.

The danger of coal mining showed in the injuries brought to the stark emergency room: hand and back injuries from falling equipment, a man with crushed legs transported to the hospital on a mattress placed in the bed of a pickup truck. I saw many hands missing fingers. The men spoke of the great danger of working for small, unregulated companies. These firms would recruit a handful of men to excavate a single seam of coal through narrow shafts with low ceilings. Sometimes these were the only available jobs.

Staff physicians worked hard and maintained a level of care equal to more affluent settings. Most of the doctors had worked for the United Mine Workers for years. Remarkably, they had avoided cynicism in these bleak and unforgiving surroundings. At supper one evening a physician a few years my senior volunteered that he served there as part of a recovery process from alcoholism. Once again I saw professionalism maintained by the insistence of physicians, not by outside pressures or inducements.

One early morning in the clinic, I called the name of a woman whose turn was next. A tall young woman in a faded sack-like dress followed me into the small examining room. Her uncombed hair was pulled into a ponytail. Her registration form stated her age as 20, although her complexion looked a weathered 40. She had a black eye; a sunken lower face dramatized already prominent cheekbones.

In a flashback I thought of Grace, in the eye of memory a strikingly similar-appearing destitute girl in my primary grades. She was retarded and seldom spoke in class. After several years in the first and second grades, the tall maturing girl was promoted each year with my class. She wore dresses of flour sacking and had no shoes. One day in sixth grade Grace did not appear. Our teacher told us that she had been taken to Millegeville, the state asylum. She never reappeared. Several of the girls in my class cried that day.

Closer examination of the Grace look-alike showed large fresh bruises on her shoulders and arms. She had no teeth. She had been beaten by her husband two days earlier.

"He whipped me."

Her answers were mumbled and sparse. Her request was simple, she wanted a new set of dentures. Following marriage at 14, she had borne four children. Her husband worked in the mines intermittently and drank whiskey each evening. She felt constantly exhausted; the thought of more children frightened her. Months earlier, she had secretly obtained birth control pills from a nurse in this clinic. Her husband was fiercely opposed to any type of contraception, so she had kept her medication hidden.

During the fateful evening her inebriated husband found the plastic packet of pills as he rummaged through her belongings. While the young children screamed and retreated for safety, he stomped the container to smithereens. He slapped his wife hard across her face, dislodging her dentures, then threw her to the floor before smashing her dentures to bits with his booted feet. Her teeth had been one of her few prideful possessions, allowing her to smile without embarrassment, and now they were reduced to pink and white shards.

She fled with her children to her people. The sheriff had been called and her husband was now behind bars. She did not know if she would press charges, however, because she could not afford his imprisonment.

She spoke in a flat, low tone, never sobbing, but tears continued to course down her cheeks. In addition to a new set of dentures, she wanted a prescription for oral contraceptive pills.

At the end of the visit a social worker promised help for the young mother and her children.

I never returned to that place after my two-week assignment. The poverty and destitution of spirit equaled that of the racial ghettos of my west Georgia boyhood. Only the color of the victims' skin differed. Both populations had been effectively sequestered within their own country, unable to pierce an invisible barrier that restricted their access to our nation's promised "liberty and justice for all."

The work of this nation is far from finished.

MOONLIGHTING

Both men had enjoyed far too many beers as they fished on the big lake. The bright sun had cooked their skin to deep red. One had the treble hook of a fishing lure stuck firmly in his external ear. His companion had two treble hooks from a gaudy bass plug imbedded in his scalp. Strands of fishing line dangled from the artificial bait. An equally intoxicated friend brought the two hooked fishermen to the hospital. They seemed oblivious to any pain.

For this challenge I recalled advice from a Boy Scout manual. After cleansing the pierced areas and infiltrating Novocain, I advanced the barbs through the skin, clipping off the points and barbs. The abbreviated hooks slipped easily from the ear and scalp of the fishermen. Neither man could explain exactly what had happened. As their euphoria began to fade into hangover, I gave each a tetanus booster and a prescription for penicillin. They left to face the rigors of alcohol withdrawal and the presumed ire of their spouses, while I addressed the needs of the next patient to sign into the community ER.

Work by Army physicians at the Elizabethtown, Kentucky, emergency room during off-duty hours had the unofficial blessing of the hospital commander. Perhaps a certain tone of goodwill with that nearby community resulted from our presence at the busy facility. For physicians needing extra money, the job was perfect, $120 for a 12-hour shift. Practice in a civilian setting was appealing. We did not have to salute anyone or wear a uniform. For an evening or a Saturday or Sunday each week we could work without fear of breaching some military code. The emergency room was well staffed. We enjoyed easy camaraderie with the nurses, attendants, and clerks. Quite competent physicians in the community were minutes away when we encountered complex illness or injury.

Sometimes military personnel sought care at the civilian emergency room to conceal events that might jeopardize their careers. One night an anxious young couple brought their crying, one-year-old son for examination. They reported the infant had fallen from his highchair and had injured his leg. X-rays showed a nondisplaced fracture of his femur and evidence of older bony trauma as well. I called the Fort Knox emergency room and learned of another visit for treatment of trauma some weeks earlier. I reported my suspicions to both military and civilian police. Two months later the nurse in the E-town emergency room told me that the baby had been brought back to the hospital, but this time he was dead. I could establish no further details of the tragedy.

Another visit by an infant had a happier ending. The young couple had taken their infant son to the Fort Knox ER earlier in the day because of fever and fussiness. Because the wait was long they returned home before seeing a doctor. They planned to treat their child symptomatically. By evening the child's fever rose higher and he cried incessantly. The baby's neck was rigid. My spinal tap confirmed meningitis, from which he made a happy and complete recovery.

During my final day of moonlighting—a Saturday—in the E-town ER, I treated the usual array of illnesses and trauma. At midnight an obese lady arrived groaning and in the final stages of labor as she was wheeled into the treatment area. She had no physician nor had she had any prenatal care. The baby's head was visible at her fully dilated cervix. There was no time to take her to the maternity ward, and besides, I was the only physician in the hospital.

She shrieked as her feet were placed in stirrups. The nurse yelled "Bear down!" I hoped I could remember the rudiments of care from my last delivery years earlier in medical school. Perhaps, like typing, child delivery is never fully forgotten. In any event, an intact, squalling baby appeared in my gloved hands. I had not needed an episiotomy; there was no tear of the mother's perineal skin.

To my surprise, where there should have been a placenta, another head appeared and I guided a second boy into the world.

Shielded from the mother by drapes, I announced, "Congratulations. You have twins."

"Goddammit," she replied. "What am I going to do with two?"

And I was never to know.

CHATTANOOGA

1971-1997

BASEBALL has woven a long and circuitous thread in the fabric of my life. My first glove bore the embossed autograph of Monte Pearson and dwarfed my hand. Boys learned the game in adult paraphernalia. Next came a Marty Marion model with a deeper pocket, followed by a Mickey Mantle outfielder's glove. My most recent anonymous, long-fingered glove is a veritable scoop of fly balls and ground balls compared to those earlier, cruder styles.

Mel Allen called the Mutual Broadcasting System's "Game of the Day" from memory's edge onward. In the pre-Muzak era of background sound it was his voice that was most likely to be heard during summertimes in the barbershops and hardware stores of small-town America. Conversation ceased within the circle of listeners at each site.

At least one Atlanta radio station indulged in sleight of ear with its detailing of away games played by the Atlanta Crackers. The announcers remained in Atlanta whenever the team was on the road. Play-by-play reports depended upon the broadcasters and their engineer improvising sounds of the action as reports of each play were delivered to them by wire. The rapt listeners in my grandparents' living room had no doubt that the announcers were in the broadcast booth of each city and that the report was instant, uttered as balls struck mitts or bats.

One evening, the announcers were unaware that the microphone was live as they talked of the ruse. Our faith in sportscasting was injured, but only for a little while.

Television intensified the drama of baseball. Before receivers were widely available, community appliance stores drew crowds to their windows during World Series time. In college not much of academic value occurred during the September championship games. When Don Larsen pitched the only perfect Series game, for the Yankees against the Dodgers in 1956, even the usually inflexible professor of my physical chemistry lab halted the class so that we could watch the epic on a small black and white set placed among the postponed experiments.

Such was the depth of talent in baseball that even semiprofessional teams provided sparkling play. I saw teams sponsored by rival cotton mills in Gainesville, Georgia, play with a ferocity suggesting that life and family honor hung in the balance. The New York Yankees supported a farm team in LaGrange. I missed few home games. At one game the home plate umpire staggered to the plate, obviously inebriated. After a brief animated conference at home plate police removed the umpire and his replacement was recruited from the stands. Another time, play was halted until a ball driven over the right-field fence—the only remaining ball fit for play—could be retrieved. In the several years of the franchise only one player ascended to a major league team and he was too old by that time to have much of a tenure.

Memorial Stadium in Baltimore provided wonderful respite from the angst of medical school. An upper deck seat cost a dollar fifty. We watched the former St. Louis Browns, now relabeled the Baltimore Orioles, begin a slow climb to respectability with a pitching staff of Steve Barber, Milt Pappas, and the veteran Robin Roberts. Once, on Bethlehem Steel Night, the great relief pitcher, Hoyt Wilhelm, rode in from the bullpen in an enormous diesel tractor. Even in this time of yearly roster re-engineering, the Orioles command my loyalty.

Chattanooga's baseball pleasures are more sublime. Engle Stadium is named for a former team owner who is alleged to have traded a struggling player for a turkey. The classic stadium provides perfect, up-close vantage points for the Class AA action. Camels parade before each game. A miniature locomotive hisses and whistles from behind the scoreboard whenever a Lookout hits a home run. We watch young players not yet spoiled by huge, multiyear contracts on the way up, and occasionally see a celebrity player working through a rehabilitation assignment. In 1995, during his hiatus from professional basketball, Michael Jordan played for the Birmingham Barons in our stadium. He was surprisingly tall for a baseball player, covered left field with remarkable speed, and his arm was powerful and true. He could not hit curves.

It was after the July Fourth game of that season. My wife and I took three boys, Bosnian refugees aged 8, 12, and 14, to watch the evening game and the fireworks that followed. Chattanooga has been referred to as the buckle on the Bible belt. A number of churches within the community had sponsored the relocation of Muslim families displaced to refugee camps by the brutal civil war that tore apart former Yugoslavia. The fathers of many of the families had been murdered or simply disappeared. Our companions represented three different families.

We watched the fireworks, leaning against our car in a parking lot across the street from the stadium. As the brilliant colors unfolded and explosions resonated, the boys drew close and the youngest held tightly to my wife. Haltingly, they spoke of the explosions of artillery and the flames from their torched homes.

The family of one had been given but 20 minutes to gather a few possessions before eviction. From a nearby farmhouse, which later was itself to burn, he watched smoke and flames pouring from his own house. People had stepped over bodies in the hurried evacuation of another village. There had been long journeys by bus; endless delays, loadings, and unloadings; and extortions by corrupt drivers.

The family of another of the boys had hidden for a time, hungry and thirsty, in a cellar before resuming their trek. His father, who had been captured earlier, had been reported terribly hurt and then killed.

We told them that they were safe now.

A nation of immigrants celebrates its independence each year. On that evening following a baseball game in Chattanooga, Tennessee, the newest members of our nation spoke simply of what the occasion symbolized. America must stand in opposition always to persecution and in support of human dignity and freedom. Anti-immigrant rhetoric that has marked debate in Congress stands as blasphemy to this founding ideal.

On summer nights the Chattanooga Lookouts play to large crowds while the city's Bosnian Americans work hard and prosper in their new home.

LORD RUSSELL'S
AUTOBIOGRAPHY

Why Bertrand Russell? The answer was to prove elusive for years. Lord Russell's principal notoriety during the years of my training derived from his staunch opposition to war and his equally fervent support for nuclear disarmament. There was no middle ground between those who denounced him as a Communist and others who revered him as a champion of individual liberty. Lord Russell's boundless energy had generated simultaneous careers as mathematician, philosopher, social critic, and writer. He received the Nobel Prize for literature. He died three years prior to his role in the life of my patient.

Margaret had moved to Chattanooga from California at age 50. Recently widowed, she chose to relocate with her eight-year-old son to a community long inhabited by her only sister, who was several years her elder. Because I already served as the physician for her sister and brother-in-law, it was only logical that I assume this responsibility for Margaret.

At age 45, Margaret had detected a lump in her breast. It was 1968. Radical mastectomy had been followed by extensive radiation therapy at a prestigious cancer institute near her West Coast home. The skin over her right chest wall sustained severe radiation injury and thereafter was to be the site of repeated breakdown, bleeding, oozing, and infection. Scar tissue proliferated and progressively distorted her arm and shoulder while tendrils of dense scar tissue stretched the skin of her neck so tightly that her head was pulled slightly askew. She consulted dermatologists and plastic surgeons and was told that nothing further could be done. She resigned herself to a regimen of daily soaks, careful cleansing of the damaged skin, and application of bulky dressings. She knew that she would need repeated courses of antibiotic therapy.

In 1971 her husband died. This ushered in the first of a number of surprises. She learned that his estate, which he had managed with great privacy, had been hollowed out by collapsing investments. He had borrowed heavily against his insurance policies and had even used their home as collateral in other leveraged deals. A further complication arose from the discovery that her husband was at least ten years older than he had alleged. Well into Social Security age, he had filed neither for retirement benefits nor for Medicare. The result of her husband's deceptions was a wickedly complicated probate, which resulted in Margaret and her son having limited funds with which to scrape by.

Margaret had taught school. Further work was out of the question, however, because of her health. Under these circumstances she determined that her safest course was relocation to Chattanooga, where she would be close to some family. She sensed at that point that her own health prospects were limited and that her son's interests would best be served by proximity to potential guardians.

She had the countenance of a refined school marm with piercing and inquiring eyes framed by wire-rimmed spectacles and lips hinting always that a smile was close at hand. Her blouse had a high-necked collar. Beneath its long sleeve, her right arm was swollen. The hand extending below the cuff was tightly edematous. Once into an examination gown, the full extent of her problem became evident. Her entire right chest wall resembled an incompletely healed severe burn. Thick crusts were interrupted by weeping, thin, reddened skin. In places, pus seeped beneath the crusts. Despite her best efforts at perfume, there was the stench of dead flesh once her dressings were removed. The skin on the front and right side of her neck was densely scarred and deeply pigmented. Other scars, which tightly constricted her right arm at the shoulder, caused the lymphatic pooling which so severely swelled her arm. She could lift the arm only with the assistance of her left hand. I worried that a thickened area behind her right collarbone represented recurring cancer.

Margaret looked over this scene of ruined flesh, seemingly unfazed as she reviewed her meticulous daily program of self-administered care. No friend or family member had ever been permitted a glimpse of her wound. We both knew that a dreadful error had been made in the administration of her radiation therapy.

Surely something could be done to alleviate her suffering. Margaret assured me that she had already run the full gamut of medical and surgical specialists before moving eastward. Nonetheless, I sought advice from an oncologist and a plastic surgeon who could suggest only minor modifications in her treatment plan.

We faced, during the next year, a slowly losing battle in which recurring infection attacked her damaged chest wall. Antibiotic-resistant strep, staph, and pseudomonas organisms thrived in her persistent wound. Miraculously, she escaped overwhelming sepsis. After initially rejecting further biopsy, Margaret consented to a procedure on the mass behind her right clavicle. Possibly this represented an infection for which some therapy might be available. The mass proved to be adenocarcinoma intermixed with dense cicatrix. Her chest x-ray showed enlarging hilar lymph nodes, which I presumed represented neoplasm. She wished to know the result of each study. She discussed the increasingly adverse finding in a logical, almost matter-of-fact fashion, reflecting for a few moments before thinking aloud.

Margaret usually came to the office alone. Twice her young son accompanied her. On these occasions when I entered the room, I would find her seated next to him reading a book aloud. She carried always a large tote bag, which contained two or three thick paperback books. When she came to the office alone, I could count upon finding her engrossed in a Jane Austen novel or a philosophical treatise. I knew only a few of the authors whom she read. We always had a conversation about books. Her commentaries were trenchant, and I added to my own personal list titles and authors whom she respected. A survey of our thoughts always followed the assessment of her wound.

In phone calls and a separate visit her sister expressed concern for

Margaret's diminishing weight and stamina. Margaret's son now spent increasing amounts of time in the home of his aunt and uncle. Margaret completed arrangements for their guardianship of her son when she could care for him no longer.

Her appetite steadily decreased. She reported almost constant nausea; eating often produced upper abdominal pain. New nodules appeared on her chest wall, obviously cancer. Some of these broke down, adding to an increasing problem of odor.

Prior to her final office visit, she requested additional time. On this occasion she stated that there was no need for examination. She had determined that she was dying and had but a few weeks left. Because of her decaying chest wall and the increasing, and finally futile, routines directed at the care of her damaged skin, she felt it best to leave her son in the full-time care of her sister and brother-in-law. She chose to enter a small, private, nursing home. She had resources that would just cover the cost, if I would promise no needless or expensive therapies.

I completed arrangements for admission to the nursing home during the following week. She had accurately predicted the more rapid decline in her health. At the time of my first visit late one afternoon after work, I found Margaret propped up in bed, quite short of breath, reading a thick paperback copy of *The Autobiography of Bertrand Russell*. Her bed bordered a window, whose ledge contained a picture of her boy and an assortment of other books. She had read, perhaps, a sixth of the way through the thick volume by the English philosopher. She had always planned to read this particular book. At the time of each subsequent visit, she had progressed a bit further in the tome.

Her son wished to visit. She chose to see him briefly in the lobby of the nursing home. She worried that he would be depressed if he saw the state of her fellow patients. Her sister told me that Margaret picked an area of the lobby where the lighting was poor so that her son would not see how sick she had become. Margaret told me of her hesitancy in giving her boy a hug, fearing he might smell the odor from her chest wall. Her sister visited Margaret daily. The sister's health, compromised by cardiac disease, became shaky from the burden of sadness that each visit generated. She could report to Margaret that her son was happy in his school and that they—the new guardians—served as parents for his homeroom.

Margaret was near the end of her book. She reviewed the content that she had covered since my last visit. She joked that God would not let her die until she finished Lord Russell's personal story. She struggled for each breath. She was reluctant to accept oxygen. She reported that pain from her chest wall was constant and no longer suppressed by Demerol.

A few days before the end Margaret was just conscious. She struggled to speak. Her fingers were blue, her breaths occurred in shallow gasps. She had completed the autobiography of Bertrand Russell. The book, in its dog-eared cover, rested on her window ledge. Despite her struggles with breathing, she was remarkably clear-headed as I sat at her bedside and held her hand.

"You finished your book."

She nodded.

She talked in staccato sentences of her son. She hoped he would go to college someday. She knew he was safe in the home of her sister. She had carefully structured her remaining resources with the aid of an attorney so that a modest trust was available to assist in her son's educational support.

"You will look in on him?"

I nodded.

Her room was almost dark as I left. She died a few days later and was buried in a private graveside ceremony.

Her son grew through his primary school years and into high school and beyond. His work was distinguished throughout. He graduated from college. His new parents, though much older than his mother, overcame their own limitations of health and participated in the full array of duties and activities for their young nephew. They cheered him in sports. They agonized when, with his new driver's license, he drove away for his first unchaperoned night out. They worried that their disciplinary demands were too strong for this child of the '70s. Should they make extra allowance in his behavior because of his loss of both parents? What was reasonable? They gave him their best efforts.

The biological and adoptive parents are all dead now. I do not know where the son lives or what career he pursues.

Years after Margaret's death I read in a 1969 *Encyclopedia Britannica* that Bertrand Russell was orphaned at age three. His father had wanted the infant raised as an agnostic, but this request was blocked by actions of a court. The persistent thread of the work of the brilliant scholar had been a search for a unifying logic of thought and action and morality. Lord Russell revered reason.

As I looked up from the maroon-covered encyclopedia, I finally understood.

ALICIA'S JOURNAL

I was born in 1926 in High Point, North Carolina, to poor uned-
ucated cotton mill workers. I don't remember much about living
there because we moved from there when I was about two years
old. I do remember my aunts and grandmother telling me about
my mother being ill with pellagra when I was a baby and [being]
very mean to me. They said that they would hide with me behind doors or anywhere to keep me from getting a whipping.
Anyway Mom got well and treated me better. The things I remember about living there is that I wore little blue and pink
dresses and every time I got a spot of water or anything on my
dress I had to have another on. I would pitch such a tantrum that
she had to change me and it would make Mom so angry she
would smack my face so hard it would be red for hours. ... The
next place I can remember is a little community in east Tennessee. My Dad Zeke and Mom Dora moved so much it's hard to
remember all the places.

Thus begins a journal left to me by my patient Alicia. She first
came to my office 20 years earlier because of intractable headaches and
uncontrollable hypertension. A tall, slender, licensed practical nurse,

she seldom smiled; often, she quietly seethed with an anger ready to uncoil. Her dark brown eyes warned of latent hostility. Neither facial powder nor smiles softened the lines of her countenance. At first Alicia volunteered little information. She distrusted physicians and most medical advice. She routinely challenged or denigrated my recommendations regarding changes in her medical therapy. Often, her systolic blood pressure exceeded 200 mm Hg. Repeated searches for a curable cause of her high blood pressure proved fruitless.

She scheduled her appointments for the early morning so that she might come to my office upon completion of a night shift. Her doleful eyes flashed with ire as she spoke tersely of some outrageous event from the previous evening. A patient might have cursed her or her supervisor had insulted her. The night shift at the sprawling nursing home never had sufficient staff. Fatigue and frustration drove her blood pressure higher and intensified her continual headaches. Routinely, she took a dozen or more aspirin per day. Despite her headaches she seldom missed a day of work. She smoked heavily and on nights off downed several beers. She steadfastly denied ever being drunk. Usually at the end of the office visit her blood pressure would have decreased substantially.

> Then we fell on really hard times in 1929 when the stock market crashed. After that we couldn't get adequate food to eat. ... One day Mom got hold of some pinto beans and there was no seasoning of any kind to cook them with and my brothers and I ate so many of them that we were up all night vomiting. A minister came by begging for something to eat and we always shared everything we had with anyone who might ask for food or lodging. Anyway when the preacher said grace he thanked God for the food and I'm sure he didn't think how it would sound but he said 'We thank you, Lord, for this food such as it is.' Well that didn't set so well with Grandpa and he let the preacher know it.

Her hypertension remained a problem. I used various combinations of medication, always in high doses. At times she seemed to challenge me to show that I could reduce her blood pressure. She doubted the efficacy of each new prescription. Once she asked, "Why don't you just give up?"

It seems that during the years of the depression someone was always living with us. There was George who was 16 at the time and worked part time in the store. He would steal candy bars and chewing gum and throw it to us across the fence. We kids loved it. One night at dusk a bunch of us kids in the neighborhood were playing hide and go seek and I ran and hid in the garage. George was in the garage for some reason but he grabbed me and was holding his hand over my mouth so I couldn't scream and he wrestled me to the ground and raped me. It hurt me badly. Then he said if I ever told anyone he would kill me. I never did tell it until I was 18 years old. I told my mother. I knew she thought when I broke down and started crying that she thought I was going to tell her I was pregnant but she put her arms around me and said 'What is it baby? Don't be afraid to tell me.' I told her the whole story. It made her so angry at George that she could have killed him and I am sure she bawled him out royally when she got the chance. ... I was a very shy and inhibited child even more after what George had done to me. I remember not wanting to take part in school. Such as gymnastics. I would not wear shorts and wouldn't take part in basketball at all. I would play softball if they didn't make us wear shorts. I think my father was the main cause of this. He was saying you can't wear shorts because girls and women aren't supposed to show their nakedness.

Bit by bit Alicia provided glimpses of her earlier years. Our region reveres softball; both slow- and fast-pitch leagues flourish for men and women. As a young woman, she was the star on a company-sponsored team that always placed well in the tournaments of summer. Rivalries among teams were rough, and there was never any hesitancy using a hard slide to take out opposing players. In one particular game all the beer, which had been iced down for a postgame celebration, was consumed before the first pitch. Tempers steadily deteriorated as the game progressed. A hard collision at home plate brought both teams onto the field, fists flying. The brawl only subsided after the police intervened. Each year Alicia gained all-star recognition as a pitcher and powerful batter. She told me that when she played, her bosses at the mill watched her instead of playing golf on their manicured courses.

With time, her palpable anger began to subside, although Alicia periodically arrived in a black mood and seemed ready to fight. Especially severe headaches or skyrocketing blood pressure readings led to many unscheduled visits to the office.

In each of her several job settings she felt always at the bottom of a pecking order. Because of skirmishes with her supervisor at work her job status deteriorated. Her final stop was the night shift at the county nursing home. She was charged with the care of a large census of hopelessly ill, elderly, and demented patients. She felt that the most unpleasant of nursing home jobs would always be assigned to her. "I was the one to clean up the vomit."

Sometimes, in moments of bleakness, she spoke of ending her life. Seeing any type of counselor was totally out of the question. In her estimation psychiatrists and psychologists occupied the deepest pits among the professions.

I listened, sometimes having to overlook repeated provocations or angry retorts. There were marriages, a child, and frightening scenes of domestic violence. A wartime job in the textile mills introduced her to amphetamines, which were widely used on the production lines to maintain alertness while working nights and overtime. The money was good if she could just work enough hours. After work she used gin and beer to quiet high levels of excitability.

When I was 18 years old my Dad came in drunk one day and started trying to beat up on all of us and I had all I intended to have of his abuse. I stood up to him and told him that he was not going to treat Mom and us kids that way anymore. We fought all over the house and Mom crying and trying to separate us. He following me all the way out on the back porch. I told him I was leaving and he said he was leaving. Finally Mom got us to agree to stay. I told him that if I stayed that I was going to pay room and board like other girls and buy me and Mom decent clothes and other things girls like. Up until then he would take all of my money and hand me back a dollar and a half. I cannot express the feelings I had during my life. I was downcast, dejected, cheerless, heavy hearted, and felt guilty. I don't know how I kept my sanity at times. I went on to be a good and respected nurse but I had severe hypertension.

With each visit, I learned more about her chaotic life. The stories came randomly, in brief snatches and never in any order, and I continued to listen.

When I was 13 years old and Dad had brought home some beer and got me to drink some. Then he started to make love to me and I managed to get away from him. He swore that he was just trying to show me what men would try to do to me. A likely story. But when I was a small girl he took me around to bootleggers and bought me drinks and I thought that he was being good to me by the attention he was showing me. ... When we moved to the city I was almost 18 and went to work at a mill just across the state line. I met a boy named Charlie. We went together for quite a while but my Dad didn't like him. Charlie had proposed to me but I refused. Partly because of Dad and partly Charlie was from Maine and was always making fun of Southerners. Dad made my life hell most of the time but he had his moments of kindness when he wasn't drunk.

Either her headaches diminished over the years or we reached a truce in our effort to control the pain. Her high blood pressure, though controllable, demanded multiple drugs for management. She challenged me on each new drug based upon her readings of the PDR. Occasionally, she smiled, and for that brief moment her facial features were warm and lovely.

She wanted to travel, to recapture the sense of freedom she felt when she had raced her old Hudson along Tennessee highways at 80 to 90 miles per hour. She loved to dance and to drink beer with a crowd. As she grew older the parties decreased. She had regarded herself always as unattractive. She seldom wore make-up when she came to the office and cut her black hair severely. In her 30s, recently divorced, she left the mill for a one-year course for licensure as a practical nurse. She had a vaguely formed ideal of helping the sick. She considered herself a quite competent nurse; however, she maintained a constant state of warfare with her superiors, thus limiting her opportunities for advancement.

Finally she was old enough to retire.

"They didn't give me a damn thing," she said after her final day of work.

Soon her chronic smoker's cough worsened and her sputum became blood-streaked. Densities appeared on her chest x-ray. Biopsy of a supraclavicular lymph node confirmed squamous cell carcinoma; bone and liver scans documented extensive metastases. She would not be able to travel. This time Alicia's threat of suicide was intense. Years earlier, as I had listened to her stories of chaos, moments of high comedy and profound sadness, I had suggested that she write a memoir or at least keep a journal. She acknowledged from time to time that she had made a few notes.

I urged her now to write that memoir rather than take her life. I argued as forcibly as I could that she had succeeded in building a life which, through her nursing, brought comfort to patients who otherwise would have known no kindness. She had raised her son, who had a good job. She owed it to herself to make sense out of her life's journey.

We did not speak of suicide again. Her cancer responded to nothing. Large doses of narcotics brought only partial relief from pain now generalized. She spent her final days in the same county nursing home in which she had worked.

Following her death, a nurse from the home brought to me, at my office, a brown paper bag that contained a Mead spiral stenographic pad. This was Alicia's journal, 32 pages written out on the lined pale green pages. As her story progressed her handwriting faltered, and she had difficulty following the lines of the pages.

The journal ended:

I was going to write more about life but I am getting very weak and in constant pain. Yes I have terminal cancer and my time here is not very long. When Jesus calls me home in the end will be my happiness. When I meet my Savior face to face. Now my doctor will finish this story because he knows me better than I know myself. I hope this short story will help young children because there is a way you can help yourself which my doctor can tell you better than I.

Below her signature she added, "Go to it, Doc. I would like to be a writer but I don't have a flair for it."

THE SIXTEEN-YEAR
HISTORY

"Why did they do those things to me?" She sounded her "w's" as "v's" as she meticulously enunciated English with a marked Eastern European accent.

I heard this question, almost a refrain, many times during the 16 years of obtaining a history from Lena.

She came to my office first in 1979. For many years she had struggled unsuccessfully to control severely high blood pressure and almost-daily severe headaches. Her previous physician had carefully searched for a correctable cause for her hypertension. He had prescribed the best available medications to little avail. Her headaches remained unchecked. I sensed that exasperation was the motivating factor for his referral of Lena to me. I would soon understand his emotion. She stated that her headaches were of such severity that she worried most days if she could tolerate the pain even until nightfall. "What is the use?" she asked.

Lena stated that she had been born in Poland, and her first husband had died after 20 years of marriage. Her second husband, to whom she had been married for almost a decade, had expired the year previous. Her only son lived in another city.

I asked where she had spent the years of World War II.

"In a concentration camp. I don't want to talk about it."

Her parents and three siblings had perished in captivity. A sister resided in Florida.

Lena was short, buxom, and of medium build. She had fair skin and prominent cheekbones. She had striking long blonde hair, which she kept tightly gathered in a large bun at the nape of her neck. Her eyes shone at times with anger and defiance; at such times her eyebrows lowered, and she would not blink. Quickly her lids would widen as a sustained wave of despair moved in. Often tears streamed from these eyes, sometimes silently, sometimes accompanied by deep, shaking sobs. She maintained a sense of elegance, her hair meticulously combed and braided, her blouse and skirt freshly pressed, her cheeks lightly powdered.

Possessed of the sense of perpetual optimism that pervades medical practice, I set about controlling her hypertension and headaches. I looked for fresh combinations of medications. I proposed strategies of stretching and relaxation for her headaches. I was confident of success. I could not anticipate what lay ahead for both of us.

Nothing worked. A severe headache awakened her each morning and persisted until bed time. The pain, at times, reached such severity that it provoked cries and the pounding of her forehead with her fist. She spoke of suicide. Each waking moment meant throbbing, piercing pain. I checked a CT brain scan. This was normal, as were x-rays of her neck. She declined evaluation by a neurologist and a psychiatrist. "They can't help me." Her blood pressure remained markedly elevated.

Her appointments were interspersed with urgent, impromptu visits occasioned by worsening head pain and her fear that she was having a stroke. Skyrocketing blood pressure readings obtained in shopping malls and drug stores caused her to panic. My nurse listened to her many phone calls with far more patience than I could muster. My every recommendation failed. I dreaded her calls and her visits, which left me perplexed and emotionally drained. Tears, anger, despair— these were the hallmarks of her times in my office. I used every therapeutic option at my disposal. I sought to reassure her—and myself.

"Why is God doing this to me? All I wanted to do was cook biscuits."

During one visit her tears ran more freely. I urged her to tell me of her girlhood, and for a moment a curtain to her past parted.

She had actually grown up in Lithuania. Following a roundup of Jews by Nazi invaders, she had been sent at age 19 to a prison camp in Poland near Cracow. She spoke haltingly of being stripped and of the coarse fingers of her captors thrust into her vagina in search of hidden diamonds. Humiliation was public and complete. Many of the captive women had their heads shaved. She treasured her long blonde hair, which she kept tightly braided and concealed beneath a cap that she wore constantly. She spoke of standing naked in a line before a low building in which she knew she would be killed. Her hair, now unfastened, draped over her shoulders. Just before she was forced into the death chamber a German officer pulled her from the line by her hair, and she was spared.

She could go no further with her narrative.

I honored her silence. I struggled to understand this story I had been given. I felt choked and heavy as I held her hand. During my boyhood I had followed avidly the events of the war with Germany and Japan. The daily radio and newspaper accounts stimulated a lifelong passion for the histories of that conflict. Of all the tragedies of that terrible struggle, the Holocaust troubled me most. Anne Frank's poignant diary placed a personal face upon the dates and statistics. I read of the hopeless uprising by the Jews of the Warsaw Ghetto against the occupying Nazi Army. Janusz Korczak, the Polish pediatrician and protector of orphans in the ghetto, became a personal hero. On the day when the Nazis evicted Korczak and the orphans from their desolate refuge to transport them to Treblinka, the doctor and his inspired charges had marched behind their personal banner to the train that would take them to the death camp. Lucy Dawidowicz's book, *The War Against the Jews: 1933-1945,* stunned me with its account of that black chapter in 20th century history.

Now a survivor of that war sat before me.

She remained firm in her refusal to see a psychiatrist or religious counselor. I sought advice from a rabbi and a Methodist minister. I asked a psychiatrist how I might proceed, which medications might best alleviate Lena's crushing depression. From my reading I learned of the guilt sometimes experienced by the survivors of overwhelming catastrophe.

The curtains to her personal history were to remain closed for a time. She agreed to a trial of antidepressant medication, which did not seem to help. We maintained our efforts to control her blood pressure and to lessen the daily pains in her head. Once, after a morning of particularly intense pain, she spoke of life's futility. She could not go on. She would kill herself. I countered that if she killed herself the Nazis would have won, that perhaps God depended upon her to be a witness to history, a reminder that mankind must eschew cruelty forever. I used this argument repeatedly at other low moments. She seemed to ponder my words.

Lena developed severe, exertional chest pain. Reluctantly, she agreed to a cardiologic consultation. Subsequent cardiac catheterization was entirely normal. She complained of increasing pain in her back and most of her joints. I suspected that years of malnutrition contributed to the osteoporosis and osteoarthritis that now progressed. Once, she agreed to see a neurologist regarding her headache. The new recommendations did not help her. She continued to hurt.

Lena left her home to shop, to visit my office, and to attend weekly services at her synagogue. She was reluctant to visit her son. She told me that he knew little of her past. When she visited him and his family she felt almost afraid to laugh or to enjoy herself. Both her son and her sister in Florida offered her living space in their homes or assistance in locating an apartment for her in their home cities. I met her son and her sister when they visited Lena during her hospitalization for chest pain. They loved her and felt frustrated in their inabilities to comfort her.

Her scheduled 15-minute visits frequently stretched to 30 or 45 minutes. Sometimes after an office visit with Lena my own head ached and I was exhausted. My nurse, after checking Lena's blood pressure, often sat with her in quiet encouragement and consolation.

The years eased by. Lena, despite unchecked hypertension, avoided stroke and cardiac problems. She achieved a truce of sorts with her vascular headaches. A fall in a store worsened her joint pain and, for a while, intensified her despair.

She agreed, after much hesitancy, to recognition in a special Holocaust memorial service at her synagogue. The years following her escape from the death house remained a blank.

She telephoned one afternoon. She wept. She had indescribable pain in her head. She had to be seen.

When I entered the examination room, she sat slumped forward. She had cut much of her hair. She had visited her niece who was hospitalized in another city because of a malignant brain tumor. When Lena had entered the room she had been overwhelmed by the sight of her niece whose scalp had been shaved.

Tears fell to the floor as Lena spoke of the war years.

In the first prison camp, she had been pushed and pressed into the low, severe building—a gas chamber. Those about her were screaming and sobbing and many vomited. Just then the door had opened. A German soldier grabbed Lena by her hair and pulled her from the room of horror. She paused for several moments before resuming her narrative. She was in another camp near the end of the war, this time huddled on the rough floor of a stablelike structure with several other weak and starved women. She was covered with rags or a blanket. She was cold and shivering. Her disheveled blonde hair was frozen to the floor, and she could not raise her head. As she drifted in and out of consciousness she was aware that her companions were led away. She recalled great noise and gunfire and then quiet.

After an interval of hours or perhaps a day, she had a vision of God on a large gray horse. "God" turned out to be a Russian soldier. He knelt over her and used his knife to cut her hair loose from the floor to which it was frozen. He wrapped her in blankets and carried her some distance to another building. She remembered a warm bath. She was weak and sick for a long time thereafter.

Throughout this story, spoken hesitantly, her tears dripped to the floor between us. Her head remained bowed.

"Why did they do those things to me?"

I understood, imperfectly, why Lena had finally cut her own hair. This act at the hands of the Russian horseman had saved her own life. Perhaps her act might spare the life of her niece.

Lena was immobilized by despondency. She could no longer bear to live. I insisted upon hospitalization and consultation with a psychiatrist. This time she consented. Her son and sister visited. After the stay in the hospital her headache diminished. She visited the psychiatrist several times. She consented to her son's overtures to relocate to a retirement home in her son's home city. I never learned what argument finally prevailed in Lena's decision to move.

I telephoned Lena a year later. She told me that she still had headaches and she took her medications for high blood pressure and depression daily. She had established some friendships in her new setting. We exchanged greetings for our religious seasons.

I had been given brief looks into a life of profound and palpable tragedy. I have yet to learn what transpired between the rescue from the gas chamber and her near death in the stable. I knew little about her early years in America. In a sense I had to connect the dots of isolated episodes to make a logical picture of Lena's life. Fear, unremitting cruelty, and starvation burned deep and permanent scars into memory which could not be shut down.

My 16 years with Lena were privileged and sacred ones. The lessons were many:

From a physiologic standpoint, severe hypertension and intractable migraine are the frequent results of overwhelming pain or grief repressed deep in memory.

Courage may manifest itself in the simple act of getting out of bed each day and proceeding through that day without being cruel to others or injurious to oneself.

We physicians do not take medical histories so much as we receive them, and this means that we must create between our patients and us an unhurried climate of trust and respect.

Continuity of care is absolutely critical if we are to understand our patients and their problems. There are limits to what we may delegate to others.

We caregivers must be comfortable with silence and, indeed, learn that shared moments of quiet reflection may enhance our understanding of one another.

I hope to visit her sometime soon.

HOW MAY I HELP YOU?

His office was half a block away. We both liked pimento cheese sand-wiches, which were made especially well at the soda fountain in the drugstore that occupied the ground floor beneath his office. We talked at least weekly, perched on the stools at the lunch counter. He was 30 years my senior. Many of my patients, their children, and their grand-children had been under the care of this legendary pediatrician.

Had Norman Rockwell met him, he would surely have incorpo-rated this doctor into a cover for *The Saturday Evening Post*. He had sil-ver hair, combed flat. His wire-framed glasses rested one third of the way down his sharply etched nose. His eyes spoke of curiosity and kindness. A hint of bemusement shaped his lips. He always seemed de-lighted to see me. I suspected this was the mood in which he greeted each parent and child who entered his office. Sometimes he wore a starched white coat, sometimes a suit jacket. His shirts always seemed perfectly starched, and his tie was never out of place. If he was stand-ing in a line-up of random males, I would predict that 90 percent of judges would identify him immediately as the pediatrician.

His stories were magical, reflecting a medical history of our place. He spoke of polio epidemics that would fill a ward with children and young people in iron lungs. He had treated typhoid and diphtheria, had seen pellagra and hookworm.

Many years earlier, at the end of a busy day, a roughly dressed man had appeared in his office.

"Are you the baby doctor?" the visitor inquired.

The man spoke of a patient in need. The doctor drove at nightfall, following the man's car to the shore of the Tennessee River where a rowboat awaited to take physician and man to an island in midstream. The doctor worried, too late, that he had been duped and that likely he would be robbed and killed. The boat landed and his companion led him to a small tumbledown shack illuminated by a kerosene lantern. Inside a lady groaned, far along in labor. Her husband had fetched the "baby doctor" to deliver this baby.

The doctor studied the situation. The lady's labor was too far advanced to correct her presumed husband's misinformation and, besides, he might never understand. Transport of the lady to hospital was out of the question. The "baby doctor" delivered the baby, a healthy child in that unhealthy and impoverished hovel. The husband had cautioned the doctor during the delivery to be careful in how he "looked on" his wife. The doctor instructed the new mother in the care of her newborn. The father paid the doctor a few dollars before rowing him back to shore.

Each year the doctor attended a reunion of his medical class. At the 60th reunion only a handful of graduates remained to celebrate the occasion. Years earlier the class had purchased an expensive bottle of brandy, which would be opened by the final survivor of the class as a kind of tribute to shared experiences. Only three alumni attended the reunion of the following year.

After retirement from practice in his mid-70s, he worked as a volunteer in the public hospital's clinic for well babies. Finally, he could no longer cope with 13- and 14-year-old mothers who brought their children for examination. They seemed to disdain any advice he tendered for the safe upbringing of their children. So he retired, again.

I felt honored when he asked, almost casually, if I would serve as his physician. When he would appear in the waiting room of my office, invariably one or more other adult patients would approach and greet him, identifying themselves as former patients. These patients in their subsequent conversations with me spoke of the repeated, loving care given to them by the pediatrician.

A severe pneumonia almost ended his life. A long-time bad knee and other joints damaged by age made it harder for him to get about.

For several years he and his wife resided in a multistoried retirement condominium. While there, he served as the attending medical advisor for the other residents. Calls for his help came throughout the day and night. He never evinced any resentment over these interruptions of his own retirement. Once he laughed as he described a previous Saturday evening in which he had been summoned to see an infant great-grandchild who was visiting one of his neighbors. A short time later, he responded to a call from a 100-year-old lady who was short of breath.

As the strength of the doctor and his wife diminished, they moved to an apartment adjacent to a nursing home. Weakness and recurrent strokes necessitated his placement in the nursing home where his wife spent most of her waking hours at his bedside. In the early months he could recognize me and we could chat about a host of topics. He realized that he would never be able to attend another reunion of his medical school class. He was uncertain if such a reunion would ever occur again. He did not know what would happen to the bottle of brandy.

During his final months he slept most of the time. When I would awaken him, his face would immediately brighten, he would smile and ask, "How may I help you?" He remained a gentleman in the waking moments that remained in his life. He had always helped by listening, by never being rushed, by extending a warm and abiding optimism that reassured all of us that we would be just fine.

JURY DUTY

And so, in 1996, I was summoned to jury duty in Hamilton County court. The state legislature had earlier enacted a law that ended the exclusion of physicians, clergy, and others from service on juries. I was to be paid seven dollars per day and could purchase my lunch from my stipend.

On the appointed Monday I joined a room full of prospective jurors. The male panelists were dressed in suits and knit shirts and overalls and khaki uniforms with name patches, which said "Buddy" or "Al." The female panelists wore dresses and slacks and tee shirts commemorating stock car races or concerts of rock and country musicians. The tee shirt of one lady was covered with Biblical quotations.

Several of the women carried young children. Perversely, I thought of a "rent-a-baby service," which would lease children to women called to jury duty so that they might claim a maternal exemption.

The clerk called us to order and announced that any excuses from service should be presented. A long line immediately formed, and from my front row perch I heard varied pleas: a sick baby, a hospitalized parent, a boss who would not understand, a pending trip out of town. Except for the women carrying young babies, the pleas were rejected.

A judge in his robe appeared and reviewed briefly the role of the jury in our legal system. He thanked us for our time and urged us to take our work in the court seriously.

I was part of a panel sent to a courtroom to hear a civil suit. From the group of 30, I was 1 of 12 selected for the jury box. During the questioning by prosecuting and defense attorneys, each of us gave a brief description of our work and activities. I was aware that a slight, tanned, and mustached, 40ish man stared at me from the opposite end of the jury box. I was dismissed from the panel. The man seemed to nod to me as I walked past him.

The following morning I joined another panel. This time I recognized from the previous day several people, including the man who had stared at me. Again the attorneys directed a variety of questions at us. This time I passed muster. The man with the stare joined me in a jury of 12. Following preliminary testimony in a case regarding a plumbing contract, we recessed for lunch. After a hurried sandwich I relaxed in the bright sunshine on the courthouse steps. The man hesitantly approached me.

"I couldn't help hearing that you were a doctor," he said.

"That's right," I said.

"What kind of doctor?" he asked.

"An internist," I replied.

"Maybe you could help me. It's my little man."

I wondered if his child was ill. Did he need the name of a pediatrician or of a children's clinic? Did he have a son or brother with growth retardation?

He continued. "It won't stand up anymore, and my old lady is pretty upset about it."

I worked hard to stifle a smile.

"Tell me more," I said.

"You see, it's been like this ..." and he outlined his dilemma. For months he had been impotent. He maintained an intense desire for sexual intercourse with his wife. His wife shared this desire. She was becoming increasingly impatient with his failed attempts at lovemaking. She questioned if there was another woman in his life.

He pulled hard on his cigarette. His tar-stained fingers reflected long-term addiction to smoking tobacco. He repaired diesel engines. To my question, he acknowledged that he might drink a bit too much: a six-pack of beer nightly, two on Saturdays. At his wife's urging he had consulted his physician, but once in the doctor's office he was too embarrassed to raise the question of impotence, which gnawed at his male identity.

In a few minutes we were due to return to the courtroom. I suggested that sometimes excessive smoking and beer might interfere with erections. Perhaps he was too tired to have intercourse. Did he ever consider spending a quiet weekend in the Smokies with his wife?

I knew his physician, a thoughtful family practitioner. I recommended an appointment specifically to address the question of impotence. If that were not feasible, I volunteered to call his physician on his behalf to alert him to the reasons for a forthcoming visit by his patient.

"I'll have to think about it. I was hoping there was some kind of prescription you could give me."

The conversation ended at that moment as we re-entered the courthouse.

A mistrial was declared and our jury was dismissed. The man and I were directed to different panels, and I did not serve with the worried man again. Once during the remaining days in the courthouse we exchanged glances across a crowded assembly room. Pocketing the several dollars not spent for soup and sandwiches, we went our separate ways.

Months later my wife and I attended an annual musical festival staged on the banks of the Tennessee River. The crowd, greater than usual, milled around food stalls, beer stands, and three huge outdoor stages. As I stood before one of the performance stages listening to a bluegrass group, I had the sensation that someone was staring at me. Turning, I saw my fellow juror standing some distance away. He wore a Western hat dotted with multiple pins and buttons. He was smoking. He raised a large cup of beer in a toast and grinned broadly before turning to disappear into the twilight audience. I have not run into him again.

Some encounters with patients—and I define the term as referring to anyone who seeks medical advice or attention from a health care professional—are curiously random. Sometimes in the face of an emergency I am called upon simply because I am the only physician present. Once, on a flight from Europe, I was summoned to evaluate a Lebanese man with the most severe urinary blood loss I have ever encountered. The stewardess and I stopped his bleeding with ice bags applied to his lower abdomen. Another time, at the YMCA, I was the only physician available to respond to a cardiac arrest on a handball court. Following the victim's recovery, he joked that I came to the "Y" solely to scavenge for patients. Other times, away from hospital and office, I am sought out by strangers with complaints of the most intimate nature. Perhaps at such times I offer the safe anonymity of a call-in show on radio.

Despite the open sexuality in American popular entertainment, we remain as individuals quite shy and inarticulate in seeking help for sexual problems. The performers in the hormonally driven offerings of television and movies stimulate expectations of erotic bliss that real people with mortgages, multiple jobs, and exasperations cannot attain. My fellow juror had branded himself a failure. Pride and shame restricted his search for answers. His complaints, haltingly presented to me on the courthouse steps, merited respectful attention.

Perhaps the broad smile of the Western-attired man whose name I never knew reflected a breakthrough in his relationship with his wife so that they could rejoice that they had found each other. I fully expect to meet him again in some unanticipated setting.

BOB'S CONCERT

Bob could easily have spent his final years in cynicism or despair. Instead, the wisdom and optimism and spiritual trust so characteristic of earlier times remained his guiding principles, even amid multiple misfortunes.

Bob had been a much-admired professor of religion and philosophy at his hometown university. His fairness in particular was praised as he resolved complex disciplinary matters involving students. His lectures were noted for their scholarly content and his examinations for their toughness.

Retirement ushered in a sequence of illnesses. Worsening angina led to a multivessel coronary artery bypass. A fall fractured his femur and necessitated an orthopedic surgical repair. Each time he pursued rehabilitation relentlessly, reading and thinking just as actively as during his career in the classroom and library.

One evening his daughter, a lovely young woman in her 20s, sustained a devastating closed head injury in an automobile accident. Although she could smile and establish for brief moments eye contact, she was to remain incommunicative and in need of continual nursing care. For years Bob and his wife, who was a pediatric physical therapist, cared for their daughter at home, until finally their efforts simply became exhausting. The young woman was to survive several more years in a nursing home.

At 76 Bob complained of steadily progressive weakness. A skeleton worn by arthritis ached diffusely. He was pale and his blood counts confirmed severe anemia. A bone marrow aspiration showed sheets of primitive malignant cells, which displaced the normal populations of white and red cells. Special stains suggested the cancer arose from his prostate gland. X-rays of Bob's skeleton demonstrated widespread bony metastases. Nothing would check the rapid progression of the malignancy.

Bob and I discussed his prospects. He did not wish any experimental therapy nor did he desire evaluation at an out-of-town oncology center. He showed neither panic nor dismay when we discussed his prognosis. His reflective calmness was the same that he would have employed in considering a problem in a philosophic text. He wished to remain at home. He charged me with control of his worsening pain.

After one visit to his home he gave me a book by Garry Wills, *Reagan's America: Innocence at Home.* We had shared many conversations about politicians and their foibles. He knew that I would enjoy this volume. He hoped that medication for his pain would not dull his intellect.

His wife tenderly and expertly cared for him in the same fashion that the two of them had ministered to their injured daughter. Husband and wife acknowledged Bob's short life expectancy; neither evinced despondency.

Bob's favorite perch was the chaise lounge in a room overlooking his home's driveway and entrance hall. There he could read, listen to music, and follow the comings and goings of friends and family. He acknowledged that his pain was worse and that simple movements were now difficult.

On my last visit as I approached the door I saw Bob propped up, wearing pajamas, his lap and legs covered by a blanket, his right hand rhythmically moving a conductor's baton. Muffled strains of Bach drifted outside. As I knocked and entered the powerful orchestral chords boomed from Bob's stereo while he conducted. After a few more bars, he interrupted the concerto with a press of a button.

A STATEMENT OF FAITH
from
ROBERT C. MILDRAM
JUNE 18, 1987
7:30 P.M.

OPENING ORGAN VOLUNTARIES

Fugue in E-Flat (*St. Anne*)	J. S. Bach
Pastorale in F Major	J. S. Bach
Christ Lay in Death's Bonds	J. S. Bach
Rejoice Together, All Ye Christians	J. S. Bach
Arioso in A-Major	J. S. Bach
Jesu, Joy of Man's Desiring	J. S. Bach

THE BURIAL OF THE DEAD: RITE ONE
Book of Common Prayer, page 469

HYMN 376   "Joyful, Joyful, we adore Thee"   *Hymn to Joy*

OPENING SENTENCES

OLD TESTAMENT LESSON—Psalm 25:6-9
    Psalm 121 (*read responsively*) page 473
NEW TESTAMENT LESSON— Revelation 21:2-7
    Psalm 23 (*read responsively*) page 476
HYMN 690   "Guide me, O Thou great Jehovah"   *Cwm Rhonda*
THE GOSPEL—John 14:1-6

THE COMMUNION

He Shall Feed His Flock	G. F. Handel
Panis Angelicus	C. Franck
Ave Verum Corpus	W. A. Mozart
Largo from Xerxes	G. F. Handel
Be Still My Soul	J. Sibelius
O Rest in the Lord (Elijah)	F. Mendelssohn
Thanks Be to Thee (Arioso in C)	G. F. Handel

PRAYER AND BENEDICTION   page 486

HYMN 207   "Christ the Lord is risen today"   *Easter Hymn*

CLOSING ORGAN VOLUNTARY

Toccata from Fifth Organ Symphony   C. M. Widor

He was assembling a memorial concert. With his unflagging smile, he told me that, for once, his friends would have to endure the music that he loved. He spoke with great appreciation of favorite works of Bach, Handel, and Mendelssohn. He wanted my opinion of the latest news from Washington, and we both poked fun at the latest pronouncements by "The Great Communicator," Ronald Reagan.

He hurt everywhere, and the pain medication did not seem to help very much anymore. During this interval, while his wife was away from home, he spoke of her soothing touch and of her ability to move him without much pain. He marveled at her skills.

When at the end of the visit I bade him good-bye, we both sensed that this might be our final meeting. He died at home several days later.

St. Paul's Episcopal Church was filled with friends and colleagues to hear the music and scripture selected by Bob for his special evening.

Following the last strains of the Widor work, we moved to the church hall for a reception. Bob's concert had lifted our spirits; there was no visible sorrow.

Several days later Bob's wife delivered three of his bow ties to me. Like all wearers of self-tied bow ties, Bob and I feigned aloofness over wearers of four-in-hand ties or, worse still, clip-on bow ties. Once, during an early visit, he had remarked that he knew at once that I was a Democrat when I entered his examination room wearing a self-tie bow tie. I cannot help but smile each time that I wear one of his ties. And I remember his special music.

THE CANE

She accompanied her husband on each visit to the office. He leaned heavily upon his cane while she supported him from his other side. Once in the examining room, she guided him carefully to his seat and stood behind his chair.

He was 75. A big-boned man with silver hair, his joints were no longer able to cope with his considerable weight. He required a few moments after he sat down before he could respond to my greeting and inquiry of how he felt. I never witnessed a smile. His voice, like his mood, was deep with dark undertones. Time and smoking had weakened his heart, and he struggled for breath between sentences. His hands rested atop the straight, heavy, gnarled cane held between his legs.

His replies were gruff and spoken loudly, perhaps because of impaired hearing, perhaps to assert a certain dominance in our exchanges.

I was far too young to serve as his physician. He tolerated me because his own physician of many years had died and I, being relatively new to the community, was available. His wife had insisted that he come to me.

When I asked a question concerning his health, he would say, "Tell him," nodding to his wife, who would then answer my question in some detail. So the interview would proceed. Only with great difficulty and much lifting could my nurse and I assist him to an examination table. He resented our effort; consequently, most of his examinations occurred while he sat. His manner ranged from grumpy to foul. The few words he spoke were spewed in bursts, while he kept his eyes fixed upon me the entire visit. He predicted, in advance, that my prescriptions would not work. He reported side effects with the medications that he agreed to take.

The challenge with such a patient is, of course, to win him over, to establish some basis for at least neutral, if not cordial exchange. I never achieved even neutrality. Typically, a visit began with the recitation of recent symptoms and observations by his wife, a thin, reserved lady, with graying hair and fair skin. Her quiet nature contrasted sharply with that of her husband. Inquiries to the patient brought little additional information. After checking his blood pressure, heart, and lungs, I reviewed his medications. He complained if expected to return in less than three or four months. His wife and I helped him to his feet. Disdaining the offer of a wheelchair, he slowly and painfully made his way along the hallway to the exit.

One visit was different. The old man asked if I would "check [his] old lady." His wife hesitated, stating that nothing was wrong and, besides, she had no time for a check-up. Nevertheless, we scheduled time for her visit. On the appointed day her husband waited outside. She provided little information. Her answers were quietly delivered; she avoided my eyes and looked at the floor. She had osteoarthritis, and her blood pressure was mildly elevated. After listening to my recommendations, she thanked me and departed.

Some months later, when the old man came for his examination, his wife seemed even more reticent than usual. She held her head turned slightly away from me. As I stood at the end of the examination, I could see bruises over her cheek and forehead, which facial powder could not conceal.

"What happened to your face?" I asked.

"I ran into a door when I got up to go to the bathroom," she replied.

I asked, "Would you like for me to check you?"

"That won't be necessary," she said.

Another visit ended.

A few weeks later, when she came to the office for her appoint-ment, I noted old and new bruises on her left arm and neck. I asked her to slip into an examination gown. She declined. She blamed the bruises on a fall down back porch steps. The footing had been slippery.

I asked if she had experienced dizziness or vertigo. She had not. She declined further examination.

I called the couple's son, a physician in a nearby community, to ask if he had noted any problems with his mother's equilibrium when he had last visited. He reported that, from his vantage point, his mother's health had shown no recent changes.

A visit or two later, the old man seemed in a mood far blacker than before. His wife wore a long-sleeved blouse. Her muted voice seemed somewhat tremulous. There was puffiness about her eyes, and one cheek was swollen.

She denied that anything was wrong and recited, as always, her husband's complaints.

At the end of the meeting I asked my nurse to assist the old man to the waiting room.

"Excuse us for a moment, I need to talk to your wife," I explained.

Reluctantly, she agreed to remain behind. I invited her to sit. She looked impassively at the floor. I asked to examine her face, where once again powder incompletely camouflaged bruises.

"Let me see your arms," I said.

She did not resist as I unbuttoned the cuffs and rolled her sleeves upward. Multiple bruises, both old and new, were apparent on both arms. A large hematoma swelled her left upper arm. She declined fur-ther examination.

I looked at her. "Something is going on here. Is someone beating you?"

She shook her head but began to weep quietly, her head bowed, hands and knees tightly clamped together.

"Is it your husband?"

Again, she shook her head, "No."

Stymied, I urged that she let me call her son or involve a social worker from Family and Children's Service to help us.

"You mustn't tell anyone," she said.

"It is your husband then," I said.

This time she nodded affirmatively.

"With his cane?" I asked.

She nodded affirmatively once again and rose to leave.

I tried again. "You must let me help you."

She declined any assistance. She begged me to remain silent. Her husband was old and sick, and she had to care for him. Illness made him do cruel things. She could not be deterred from leaving, after seeing to her face, re-applying facial powder, and gathering her composure.

I left word at her son's office for him to telephone me upon his return from hospital duties. When he called at midday I indicated that we needed to meet to discuss a confidential and urgent matter. He was terribly busy. Could we not discuss the matter now?

I reviewed my observations for the previous two years and the denouement of that morning.

"This is a family matter. You mind your own damned business." He hung up.

I phoned the battered wife the next day. She stated that she was fine, and that she neither wanted nor needed any help. The family would take care of its own problems. She reminded me that her husband was quite ill and in need of her care. I listed ways in which she could obtain help, but she seemed little interested. She must hang up because her husband became upset if she spoke over the phone too long.

I never saw either of the physician's parents again as patients.

After a long interval I read the brief obituary of the old man. I wondered what had happened to his wife. I never saw her son or any family member from whom I could learn of her fate.

Years later, during the national debate on health care reform, I addressed a group of senior citizens on the issue. After my remarks, while cookies and coffee were passed around the room, several members of the audience pressed their questions informally. The final person to greet me was the old man's widow.

She had aged surprisingly little. Her hair had whitened. Eyes that once had reflected the fear of a deer caught in headlights now seemed calm and alert. Her speech was crisp. She remained slender and moved easily.

She thanked me for my remarks. We engaged in safe chitchat about children and grandchildren. She visited regularly among her circle of friends and was active in her church and in Senior Neighbors.

When I asked her how she had been she said, "Just fine." But as she turned to leave, she paused for a moment and asked, "You never told anyone, did you?"

I smiled, and deferred an answer. She turned away to rejoin the larger group in the social wind-down after a doctor's talk.

I know now of the pernicious extent of domestic violence. I have seen it many times and in unexpected settings. Were I to encounter the old man with a cane and his wife today, I would suspect his beatings much earlier. If the son declined intervention, I would call without hesitation the domestic violence hotline sponsored by my community's Family and Children's Service.

I wonder what became of the cane? Was it buried with the old man? Is it in the closet or garage? Was it simply thrown out?

AURORA BOREALIS

Emotional overload always lurks as a hazard to medical practice. When a patient of many years dies, I grieve; sometimes several losses occur within the same week. When I detect a rapidly progressing and incurable neoplasm in a patient, I ache and know that I must steady my voice and my emotions for the forthcoming discussion with my patient and his or her loved ones.

I find peace with my family, children, and grandchildren, with books and baseball, and with canoeing. Chattanooga is located within easy drives of gorgeous streams and rivers, perfect for day-long floats. The effect of a day-long paddle on the Hiawasee River at Reliance, Tennessee, is almost mystical.

Because of our love of the water, it was natural that Ruzha and I decided to celebrate our 30th wedding anniversary with a week-long canoe trip in Minnesota's Voyageurs National Park. One night during this excursion, quite by accident, we saw the northern lights in full display. This is how it happened.

We had canoed the area several times before with various combinations of our sons and friends. From previous trials and many errors, we had become competent in our use of maps and compass. We could pack and unpack our canoes expertly, set up a campsite, light a fire, and start food cooking in 30 minutes or less. We could paddle for hours and manage the full array of portages, which linked the many lakes. On each trip, we knew that within a day or two of paddling we would be in an area of serene beauty which, depending upon our route, might include rocky palisades at water's edge or dense groves of birch trees on gentle slopes. Sometimes, we had portaged our packs and canoes alongside chaotic waterfalls. From prior experience, we also knew that if we timed our trip for August we would not encounter the large man-eating mosquitoes that flourish throughout the lake country in spring and early summer.

For our anniversary trip we worked out an oval route that would take us into remote lakes we had never before visited. By pushing and paddling hard, we planned to make Little Saganaga Lake by our second night. We arrived late on the second day in a driving rain. However, the next day dawned and revealed a vast lake of deep blue water studded with islands. This was too pretty to leave but leave we must if we were to complete our circuit.

Our first problem began. The jagged coastline featured cove after cove, and we could not locate the entry to the portage to the next lake. We paddled for hours, taking repeated compass sightings, feeling repeatedly that the long-necked cove that we were about to enter would be the right one. Finally, in late afternoon, we were tired and wondered if we would ever find our way out of this beautiful lake which now seemed our nemesis.

Just then, the first canoe we had seen that day came within hailing distance; a red-bearded Canadian and his powerfully built wife were paddling through on their honeymoon. We explained our predicament. The groom assured us there was no problem at all. If we simply paddled north a short distance we would come to a rock covered with orange lichen. If we turned immediately leftward at that point we would be at the entry of a long cove, which would lead to our portage. By nightfall, we had made it to the next lake, and prospects for the anniversary trip were again looking up.

The goal of paddlers on those lakes is to locate the perfect campsite. These are generally placed by the Forest Service and consist of a clearing with a fire grate, a nearby box latrine, and usually a small stack of firewood left by the previous campers. Sometimes, only a single campsite will be situated upon a lake.

We found the idyllic spot: a small clearing surrounded by rocks and trees with a gentle slope ending in smooth rocks perfect for landing and unloading a canoe. The view across the open water to steep rocky bluffs was as stunning as any we had ever enjoyed in the Boundary Waters.

We had encountered black bears on previous journeys and once again took the necessary precautions of hoisting our food packs in a rope sling suspended between tree trunks that had no easily accessible lower limbs. We arranged brush and firewood so that, if needed, a blaze could be quickly started to frighten away any bear. Pitch darkness on that moonless night descended by 10:30. All was quiet.

Suddenly, we were awakened by something large and swift brushing the aluminum frame of our tent. It had to be a bear! We sprang into our routine, bursting from the tent, shouting, and aiming the beams of our flashlights toward the food pack slung high in the trees. A large black bear stood beneath our food packs, swiping at the one pack just out of his reach. He was not deterred by our light and noise. Ruzha threw a match into the dried brush beneath the grill, and we immediately had a brisk fire, which also did not deter the bear.

After surveying the ropes and food pack this bear, obviously skilled in such raids, climbed a few feet up one of the tree trunks and deftly cut the rope forming the sling. No sooner had our food pack crashed to the ground than the bear grabbed it and loped into the woods. In the excitement, I dropped my glasses and momentarily thought of the hunger I would experience during the long paddle back to our drop-off point. In that instant Ruzha pulled a fiery brand from the fire and yelling, "Come back with my food!" charged into the woods on the trail of the bear. I found my glasses and followed the light and the noise into the trees.

Perhaps 50 yards into the thicket I found Ruzha and the bear, the large animal standing on his hindquarters, his escape blocked by an embankment. He was faced by Ruzha, now flailing away at his nose with the fiery brand while beaming her flashlight full in his face with her other hand. Sparks flew.

"Grab the pack!" I reached in and snatched the pack clear, amazed in that moment how the face of that great bear, at eye level, resembled a large rat.

We bolted to our campsite, guided by the light from our fire. I heard crashings in the undergrowth behind us. I feared that the bear would return at any moment, so I set about sawing firewood to sustain a large blaze until dawn. I expected an attack at any moment from a bear unlikely to be in a good humor. Ruzha, ever trusting the ways of nature, rolled up in a tarp to sleep within the circle of light. I sawed and sawed. And then glancing skyward, I beheld it. At first I thought I must be hallucinating; I had never witnessed such a spectacle: whirls and waves of blue, green, and yellow lights advancing and receding. I felt that these had to be from footlights surrounding our site, so vivid and mobile were the illuminations. I awakened Ruzha, and we watched the kaleidoscopic show as it continued until finally it faded not long before dawn.

After breakfast and loading our canoe we retraced the bear's trail into the forest. In a rough clearing at the foot of the embankment were shredded remains of other packs and scattered, torn wrappings of freeze-dried food belonging to campers less fortunate than we. We pushed off for the remainder of our anniversary journey, which was relaxed and uneventful.

In that space of nature were all of the elements of so many clinical encounters. There was fear and uncertainty and the pragmatic and feeble responses of human beings against wilder, potentially more powerful forces of nature. When we were tired and lost on an unfamiliar lake, knowledgeable strangers calmed us with a gift of clear directions. At our tent site momentary despair was reversed by bold action, and there was, at the end, almost indescribable beauty.

Illness, with all of its capacity for surprise and disorganization, places my patient and me in a metaphorical canoe launched upon uncharted waters with imperfect maps and compasses. The disease may be negotiated safely or ruined health or death may ensue. If we are lucky, my patient and I, we will perceive beauty in unlikely places before our shared journey is complete. This beauty may be a fresh insight or possibly a renewed relationship with a beloved one. We may share the satisfaction of conquering or containing an illness. These unexpected treasures may be no less spectacular than the northern lights.

A CALL FROM BOLOGNA

In the heyday of radio, "Fibber McGee and Molly" anchored Tuesday night's comedy lineup. In each episode Fibber McGee would absent-mindedly move toward his closet. Despite the warnings of wife Molly he would open the door. There followed a series of crashes, metallic bangs, tinkles, and thuds as, over the next several seconds, all that was stuffed in the closet crashed to the floor in front of the hapless Fibber McGee. Long-forgotten objects from years earlier might be pulled from the debris. Fibber McGee's closet entered our jargon as a place where clutter could safely be stashed away.

An internist's brain bears certain parallels to Fibber McGee's closet. We are inveterate clutter mongers, accumulating case histories, un-usual clinical findings, random biologic facts searching for a home, and other accumulated oddments from the very dawn of our clinical expe-riences in medical school. A physician who may struggle to recall where he might have laid his stethoscope will instantly recall a bizarre case from years earlier, recounting in precise detail the setting, the ap-pearance of the patient, and the thrill of finding an unexpected pathogen upon a microscopic slide.

In 1964, on Vanderbilt's private medical service, our team of in-terns and residents helped care for a sick physician from another state.

He suffered abdominal cramps and had lost considerable weight. He was losing his hair. Strands could easily be removed by the slightest of tugs. He complained of burning pains in his feet and weakness when he tried to walk. Our studies strongly suggested arsenic poisoning. But how? And by whom? And was this accidental or intentional?

Upon presentation of the suspected diagnosis to the physician-patient, he vehemently denied the possibility. We searched for information supportive of accidental exposure; there was none. When we asked if there might be a grudge-bearing acquaintance who might wish him dead, he irately denied this possibility. Poisoning was simply out of the question. Still upset, he checked out of the hospital and returned home. We learned of his death several weeks later. A case that was never fully opened would never be closed.

Early one afternoon in February of 1989 the switchboard operator in my office paged me. Unlike the myriad calls of every day, this one was different. It was from Italy. The call was from Peter, an American studying in Bologna. This 25-year-old graduate student had grown up in Chattanooga. After a distinguished undergraduate career at our city's university, he had been awarded a fellowship for study of modern languages at Oxford University. I had met him during the competition for this award, and we had subsequent conversations when he returned home to visit his parents.

Peter was now in his second year of study abroad. He had arranged specialized study in Italian at the University of Bologna where his call originated.

"Dr. Cleaveland, this is Peter, and I'm sick."

The voice was deep and rasping and its cadence even more deliberate than the usual Southern pace of his speech. I inquired what was wrong. He reported a 12-pound weight loss during the two preceding weeks. His appetite had failed, and he experienced nausea with each attempt at eating. His sleep had become fitful with vivid, hallucinatory dreams. His feet ached and felt swollen and numb. Any movement produced aching in his ankles and knees. His abdominal muscles ached as well, and numbness ascended from his feet to the level of his chest. When he walked he was aware that his feet seemed to flop against the floor. His weakness was progressive. Several days earlier his hair had begun to fall out.

I asked if he had seen a physician in Bologna. He had. He had been given injections, possibly a potassium compound, but these had been ineffectual. His doctor was unable to attach a diagnosis to Peter's symptoms. Peter surmised that he was terribly ill.

I advised him to return immediately to Oxford and to go immediately to the Radcliff Infirmary. In the closet of my mind, a linkage had been established.

That evening I worried. What could it be? The Oxford physicians could surely pinpoint the cause.

Twenty-four hours later Peter appeared in my office. His parents assisted him as he walked slowly along the hallway.

This was his story.

Peter had come home for the Christmas holidays of 1988. He returned to Italy in mid-January. He experienced a flu-like illness, which was treated with antibiotics. Prior to this time he had been very active, playing basketball two to three times each week.

A couple of days prior to the first symptoms of weakness and weight loss, he recalled eating dinner in the student cafeteria of his university. The main course, a meat dish, did not taste quite right. A servant brought an extra helping of meat to him after he was seated. In his student dormitory another foreign student experienced similar but milder symptoms several days prior to the onset of Peter's symptoms.

Relentlessly during the next two weeks, Peter's illness progressed. He ate several additional meals in the student cafeteria until his appetite failed.

Peter appeared chronically ill. The tall, lean, soft-spoken young man now appeared gaunt. The hair on his scalp had thinned. I could pull individual hairs free with the slightest of pulls. His blood pressure was 90/70, and he had a resting pulse of 54. His ankle extensors and flexors were weakened; otherwise, his reflexes and sensation seemed intact. I thought of the poisoned physician.

Blood counts, urinalysis, and a chemistry profile were normal. Blood lead and coproporphyrin levels were normal. I sent blood and urine specimens to our reference lab for arsenic and mercury levels.

Two days later Peter reported a metallic taste and worsening of the tingling paresthesias in his feet and ankles. He now had conjunctivitis. His thigh muscles had weakened.

There followed an amazing string of laboratory gaffs. After a delay and many increasingly impatient phone calls, the reference lab reported a breakdown in their analytic equipment. The blood and urine samples were relayed to another lab, which reported trace amounts of arsenic and lead.

Back to the toxicology textbook. Thallium poisoning jumped from the page. I directed Peter and his parents to Nashville, where I hoped toxicologic studies for thallium could be done with promptness and accuracy. There was further delay. My impatience grew; I was concerned for my patient.

Years earlier the toxicology laboratory at the Massachusetts General Hospital had helped me in the diagnosis and management of another patient, this time with beryllium poisoning. I telephoned the director of that division and explained my patient's dilemma and my diagnostic frustrations.

"Send him up." The great hospital had again come to the rescue.

Perhaps too many James Bond movies had influenced me. I called our State Department. After several transfers I spoke with a man who monitored violent acts against Americans on foreign soil. He consulted a computer database. There was no evidence of poisoning or other violent deeds directed against Americans in Bologna. I reported my findings to the U.S. office that directed the scholarship program which sponsored Peter's overseas study. I shared my suspicions with an investigator who called from Europe.

In the meantime Peter had been admitted to Massachusetts General Hospital, where dangerously toxic levels of thallium were detected in samples of his blood and urine. Shortly thereafter, similar confirmatory reports belatedly arrived from Nashville. I talked with Peter's resident and his neurologist. Large doses of activated charcoal would be employed in his treatment.

Peter steadily improved.

While Peter was still hospitalized, I returned to Oxford to attend the inaugural dinner of my college's medical alumni association. I paid a visit for tea at Rhodes House, which served as the headquarters for

Peter's fellowship program. The Warden, a wiry and intense former tutor, had closely monitored Peter's illness. During my visit we telephoned Boston and spoke directly to Peter, whose voice now sounded normal. I sat down for tea with the Warden and his wife. Neither had learned of the cause of Peter's disease. While tea was poured and sandwiches passed, I reviewed the strange sequence of symptoms and events. Before I revealed the diagnosis, the Warden's wife interrupted, "Why, it must be thallium."

"But how did you know that?" I asked incredulously.

She rose quickly and walked to a large bookcase, which she scanned for a few moments before retrieving a paperback copy of Agatha Christie's *The Pale Horse,* written many years earlier. She thumbed through the book in which multiple murders had occurred and several symptoms were described: hair loss, peripheral neuropathy, gastroenteritis, and difficulty speaking. She excitedly read several brief passages.

Quite clearly, a devotee of Miss Christie's mysteries would be a valuable addition to any diagnostic team.

Peter returned to Chattanooga on a continuing regimen of frequent large doses of activated charcoal by mouth. His strength gradually returned. His hair could no longer be dislodged from his scalp with ease, although months would pass before normal hair growth returned. Dense white, transverse Mees' lines marked his fingernails as they grew.

Two months after his hurried return to America, Peter left for Oxford. He would need a full year to complete his recovery.

The exact circumstances of the deliberate poisoning of Peter remain unclear. Thallium is readily available in Western Europe as a rodenticide. The rats and mice of Europe are now resistant to the effects of warfarin, which remains the most frequently used poison for such pests in our country. I received one additional phone call from abroad, from another investigator. His accent sounded more French than Italian. Other students had been identified who suffered from thallium poisoning. A kitchen helper was suspected. Apparently the felon had a hatred for students foreign to Italy. He had timed his poisonings to occur prior to a spring vacation in which the foreign students would return to their homelands, and where their illnesses might be harder to diagnose. Additional servings of thallium-laced meat had been delivered to these students at their dinner tables.

Thereafter, a veil of secrecy dropped over the entire affair, and I could learn nothing further about motives, mechanisms, or possible suspects. In a later communication the Warden assured me that no one had died.

Chance and memory played powerful roles in the diagnosis of Peter's illness. Because both unrecognized thallium and arsenic poisoning can lead to permanent intellectual impairment, seizures, or death, prompt diagnosis is crucial. Colleagues in Boston whom I have met only by telephone and mail saved the day.

SAGA OF THE
THREE SISTERS

≈

Lora Mae Cross was deeply jaundiced when I first saw her, and her belly was swollen. Her husband accompanied her to my office. They lived on a farm atop Sand Mountain in northeast Alabama. A lady in her mid-50s, Lora Mae had been vigorously active until recent weeks, managing the home and frequently helping her husband with light chores in the barn and the fields of potatoes. At first, her appetite faded; even the thought of food caused severe nausea. She steadily lost strength. She noted a darkening of her urine and a lightening of her stools. As her abdominal girth expanded, Lora Mae suspected that she had cancer. A sister moved in to care for her and to help with the duties of the household whose mistress could no longer rise from her bed.

Mr. Cross viewed physicians with some suspicion. He held strong beliefs that nature would heal any sick person if he or she was meant to survive. Reluctantly, he called a family physician whose careful initial examination suggested that Laura Mae had obstructive liver disease. The doctor telephoned me to schedule an appointment. Mr. and Mrs. Cross drove to Chattanooga the following day.

The shy and soft-spoken lady from the country was deeply jaundiced and quite ill. She seemed resigned to the fact that her remaining days were quite limited. Her liver was enlarged and granite hard. Ascitic fluid swelled her abdomen.

Reluctantly, Mr. Cross agreed to the hospitalization of his wife. He worried about the expenses which might be incurred. He urged that I do everything possible to limit his wife's stay in the hospital to the shortest time possible. The family could take splendid care of her in the home.

Laboratory studies pointed to a severe obstructive process in Lora Mae's liver. Her bilirubin was 16. Her blood ammonia level was elevated. A CT scan delineated a dense infiltrative process, thought most likely to represent carcinoma, throughout the liver.

I questioned Lora Mae and her husband closely. She was offended when I inquired if she consumed any ethanol. She emphasized that in her church consumption of alcohol in any form was a sin, and she had always honored that teaching. She had taken no medications. She could recall no exposure to potentially toxic materials on the farm. She never handled any of the herbicides or fertilizer that her husband used on his crops. She was one of three sisters, the eldest of whom had died a year earlier in a Georgia hospital of a liver ailment.

I consulted a gastroenterologist who, after his evaluation, advised percutaneous liver biopsy. He obtained a leathery, yellow core of tissue. Studies by pathologists documented diffuse, hepatic amyloidosis. A hepatologist in Nashville reviewed the microscopic slides and remarked that he had never before observed such dense deposits of amyloid. Few hepatic cells remained. There was no prospect for reversal of Lora Mae's disease.

Lora Mae returned home to die. Her daughter from Chattanooga and her surviving sister from Sand Mountain tended to her needs daily. Her rural physician documented Lora Mae's steady deterioration as we used the meager means at our disposal to keep our patient comfortable.

Mr. Cross brought his wife to my office for a final visit. In the intervening weeks her peripheral muscles had wasted away. She was even more deeply jaundiced, but she remained alert and quietly resigned to her impending death.

"I'm going to a better place," she stated.

I quizzed Mr. Cross again. Had there been any possible toxins to which his wife might have been exposed?

Again he answered, "No."

And then he remembered that he had contacted an extermination company to deal with an infestation of roaches around the cover of the well that supplied water to his house. The pest killers visited his farm repeatedly, applying at each visit a pesticidal powder at the periphery of the cover overlying his well. The applications had been successful; the roaches disappeared.

I asked that he bring me a gallon of the water for analysis. In the meantime I contacted public health officials in his home county, and they referred me to the state health department. After several transfers of my call I was directed to Auburn University, which was home for an analytic laboratory specializing in pesticide residues.

Mr. Cross returned to my office with a gallon jug of clear but, as I would learn, deadly, water. Subsequent studies by the Auburn scientists documented in the well water a concentration of the pesticide, heptachlor, far above the known toxic threshold.

With this information in hand I again contacted public health officials for the state of Alabama. My telephone calls led nowhere. The buck was repeatedly passed through a bureaucratic maze. No one seemed interested in pursuing an investigation into possible poisoning from heptachlor. I turned to the division of oncology at the University of Alabama Medical Center in Birmingham. A cancer epidemiologist listened to my story with great interest. He assembled a team to search for answers.

In the meantime, Lora Mae died. Soon afterward her remaining sister became ill. A physician at an Alabama hospital diagnosed hepatoma. The sister's health steadily worsened. When she was at the threshold of death, her husband agreed to the request of the cancer epidemiologists that immediately after her demise a large specimen of liver would be obtained to seek a link between the hepatic malignancy and exposure to heptachlor. Had the sister ingested sufficient contaminated water from Lora Mae's well to stimulate malignant change in her liver?

At the time of the sister's death, her husband had second thoughts and declined further study of his wife.

"She's suffered enough," he explained.

The epidemiologists from the University of Alabama pursued a search for carcinogens throughout the rich farming area of Sand Mountain. Soil and water samples were collected from farms whose owners were often suspicious and sometimes quite hostile to the investigators. The resulting studies uncovered a frightening pattern of soil pollution by a variety of potentially toxic agents probably disseminated by repeated aerial spraying. Those farms not served by municipal water supplies had an alarming incidence of hepatic and bladder carcinomas among their occupants.

Mr. Cross and his daughter remained well. Neither had been exposed to the well water to the extent of Mrs. Cross and her recently deceased sister.

Hospital records relating to the illness and death of the first sister were fragmentary, simply reporting rapid hepatic failure in a lady who had spent a lot of time in the home of Lora Mae.

Quite by chance, I encountered briefly another patient from a small community on Sand Mountain during this time. This middle-aged lady lived and tended a store in her hamlet. She suffered from failure of her bone marrow and she would soon die. She dated her illness from a day in which dense fog blanketed her hometown. Crop dusting aircraft, which frequently crisscrossed the potato fields abutting the town, laid down a dense cloud of pesticide that day. The choking poison hung in air until the fog cleared the following day. This lady's goldfish died; her cat was sick for days. She knew of other people in her community who had been sick since the crop dusters had flown over on that fog-bound day. She was never to feel well again and died within a year.

Had she not considered reporting her suspicions to county health officials?

She had not. She feared retribution from powerful landowners. She might lose her job.

I reported this matter, but I could never obtain much in follow-up. I did learn that the owner-pilots of the crop dusting service had themselves died of cancers.

Three sisters succumbed to liver disease within a year and a half of one another. They were close neighbors. The well of one, Lora Mae Cross, had been poisoned by men who had recklessly spread pesticide at the opening of her well. The pesticide, heptachlor, would soon be banned because of hepatic toxicity and carcinogenicity. Strong circumstantial evidence linked heptachlor to the destruction of Lora Mae's liver by deposits of amyloid. The etiology for the fatal liver problems of the other two sisters remained unsettled. Both had spent many days at the home of Lora Mae either during or prior to her illness.

Sand Mountain in Alabama is blessed with rich soil, which gives forth lush crops of potatoes and other vegetables. The mountain is dotted with prosperous farms and pleasant towns and villages. Careless and unregulated use of dangerous chemicals cast a pall of disease and death over this farming region. Local and state officials seemed uninterested. Energetic scientists from the university delineated the dangers in studies, which confirmed the hazards of heptachlor.

There are those in business and political circles who fight environmental protection at any level of government. The foes of such legislation point to the need to create jobs and to stimulate business. I saw through my experience with my patient, a kind and devout farm lady, the tip of a dangerous iceberg that continues to beg for intense scientific study and federal legislation to protect our people from poisons in the air above and the soil and water below.

MAGIC

Except for long-standing hypertension, Harris enjoyed excellent health, his only symptom being occasional fleeting palpitations. A tall and quiet man with unflappable good humor, he and his school teacher wife raised their children and then turned their considerable energies to community volunteerism.

Harris' first neurological symptoms began when he was 54 years old. He awakened, usually about 2:00 A.M., feeling anxious and as if "my motor is going too fast." He checked his pulse each time and found it to be slow and regular.

A few months later Harris slipped on ice and fell hard, separating his right shoulder and striking his head on a step. He recalled being dazed for several minutes but did not lose consciousness.

His shoulder healed, except for mild limitation of upward movement. Harris began to note in his sales work that he could no longer recall names, addresses, and orders with the speed and facility of the year before. In addition, he had to jot down notes and rely increasingly upon a secretary in his office to prompt his memory. He continued to work full-time but under a cloud of worry that he might miss some critical appointment. His episodes of feeling hyperactive became both more protracted and frequent. These might occur day or night. In between, he often felt sluggish with blunted powers of reason. His balance became mildly impaired to the extent that stairs or uneven terrain required extra concentration to negotiate.

I worried that his earlier fall on ice had damaged his brain. A brain scan, an electroencephalogram, and a carotid ultrasonogram were normal. A neurologist examined him and advised a trial of Dilantin for a possible subtle seizure disorder.

During the next eight months Harris had more problems with his memory. His notes no longer helped. His secretary had to remind him several times each day of scheduled responsibilities. In a business meeting he was aware that he could not concentrate and that details of the presentation quickly slipped away from him. He prided himself on hard work and expertise in sales. He feared that he was likely to embarrass his company in a major way and thereby lose, if not his job, then the respect of his colleagues.

The neurologist and I conferred. We referred Harris for neuropsychological testing. This detailed study documented a moderately severe amnestic disorder. For the first time Alzheimer's disease was raised as a diagnostic possibility.

His memory worsened. He was unable to remember room numbers when out of town on overnight business trips. Names of long-term clients escaped him. He could not recall a conversation with a customer if an hour or two had elapsed following a business call. Further psychometric testing and neurological evaluation increased the likelihood of Alzheimer's disease. Retirement, which Harris had planned electively for age 60, now became mandatory because of his disability.

As too often happens, the formal process of disability determination was complex, drawn out, and exasperating for Harris, his wife, and me. The disability insurer questioned Harris' symptoms and challenged my findings. Perhaps the insurers deal with too many fraudulent claims. For claimants with valid career-ending disease, the process of obtaining benefits is often demeaning. Approval of this disability claim required months of negotiation.

Throughout his diagnostic workup Harris and his wife wanted the facts laid out logically and precisely. Because of his fading memory,

Harris brought his wife to most of his examinations. Once the likelihood of Alzheimer's disease was presented, Harris convened a family conference to discuss his diagnosis and prognosis with his children. If his time of independent activity was limited, he determined that it would be as productive as possible.

Harris established a schedule of early morning workouts at a community gymnasium. After this warm-up he drove to a nearby school to work as a volunteer, reading aloud to kindergarten and first-grade students.

"This is the most enjoyable thing I have ever done," he reported to me.

Following a rest, Harris proceeded next to work with a voluntary crew dedicated to highway beautification. He dug, raked, planted, and felt a special satisfaction with the array of blossoms that transformed an otherwise stark highway intersection.

At each visit to my office he was frank and analytic. His numerical skills were no more. Without his trusty pocket-sized notepad he would forget most appointments. He knew his days of independent activity were dwindling steadily. He worried about a future in which he could no longer drive to his appointed rounds of reading and gardening.

His wife retired early from her teaching job. Their shared looks and held hands reflected an abiding love. They remained calm and mutually supportive in the face of this illness.

During a recent visit to my office Harris was more apprehensive than before.

"I haven't got much longer. I love to read to the kids. I feel like one of them."

His daughter was pregnant with a due date but a few weeks away. Accompanied by his wife, Harris had joined his daughter at the office of her obstetrician the day before. Harris had seen the shadowlike movements of the fetus, its forehead and nose and precisely defined fingers and toes.

"It was magic. It's what it's all about. I can't wait to see that baby."

Harris was concerned that it would not be safe for him to hold the new grandchild. He might drop the infant. He longed to touch ever so lightly the face seen in two dimensions on the ultrasonographic screen.

He smiled broadly as he shook my hand and wished me well.

A couple of weeks later as I drove at dawn to work, I approached the ramp which bordered the flower garden on which Harris worked. In the middle was anchored a pink balloon announcing "It's a girl!"; a friend had placed the tribute.

A few days later Harris returned to my office, smiling and unable to sit still as he described his first grandchild.

"They handed her to me, and all I could do was hold her and look at her and cry. I couldn't talk. Isn't it great?"

Once again, he shook my hand and extended best wishes for a good day.

This brave man whose illness steadily eroded the functioning of his brain, who knew that someday soon he might lose his independence and later the ability to communicate with his wife and children and new grandchild, chose a course of aggressive optimism. As the diagnosis of Alzheimer's disease became clear, he briefly was shaken and sad. Coaches speak to their teams about "sucking it up," about reaching for a high level of performance that can yet win the contest. Harris, my patient and friend, continues to exemplify what "sucking it up" really means when applied to the business of living and loving.

HERE COMES TROUBLE

No words in the 1940s struck greater fear into parents and children alike than "polio," or "infantile paralysis," as it was more commonly called. For a time, each summer season ushered in a fresh epidemic. Radio and newspaper reports described severe outbreaks in Charlotte or Atlanta or Birmingham. If a case was confirmed in LaGrange, public swimming pools closed, and we would avoid movie houses and any large public gathering.

If a child complained of headache or flu-like symptoms during summer months, parents summoned the physician immediately. All would breathe sighs of relief when symptoms remitted. Some children in my community were not so lucky. One summer, the older sister of a friend and the leader of my Cub Scout den were struck. Both required months for recovery.

The proximity of LaGrange to Warm Springs, Georgia, heightened our awareness of polio. The trips of President Roosevelt to the famed treatment facility were covered in detail by the press.

Such was the lack of knowledge of polio and its mechanism of spread that one elderly physician in my community sprayed children under his care with DDT in hopes of warding off the dread illness.

While I played and worried in LaGrange, in another town in

northern Alabama, a little girl suffered an attack of polio in its severest form. She was four years old. Thirty years later she would become my patient.

Initially, the little girl was not expected to live. On the advice of a trusted physician in her home community, her parents placed her on a pillow and took her to Nashville for further evaluation. The physician there urged her parents to leave the little girl in a Nashville hospital and forget about her; there was no hope. They took her back home. Another physician recommended the removal of her tonsils, a proce-dure complicated by a near-fatal hemorrhage. She recalls even today being so weak that she could not lift her head or her hands from the bedclothes. Her parents searched further for a physician who might give them hope. Her mother phoned the chamber of commerce in Memphis and asked for the name of the best pediatrician in the city. Her parents once again placed her upon a pillow in the back seat of their car and drove to the office of the esteemed physician. He trans-fused the little girl. Following his examination, he outlined a course of home therapy for the severely weakened child. He doubted that she would live more than a year. She would suffer less if kept in the com-pany of other children. She had no siblings. Her parents invited chil-dren of the neighborhood to be with her. A brother was born nine months later.

A visiting teacher came to the little girl's house until she was eight, when her formal education stopped. She read voraciously. If no other books were available, she read the dictionary. Because both parents worked, a country lady was hired to help her aged grandmother care for the girl during the hours when her parents were away. Her mother baked endless trays of cookies for the children whose presence lifted the little girl's spirits.

The family moved, finally settling in Chattanooga in 1960. A physician recommended severing tendons in the young woman's an-kles so that she might walk; she refused the experimental therapy.

In 1972 her mother and father pushed the wheelchair bearing my new patient into my office. Her white-haired elders stood as I entered the examination room. They introduced Mary Ruth, who smiled and extended a delicately thin hand to mine.

Her voice had the timbre of an actress. Her vocabulary was rich and her grammar precise. She explained that she had come to see me in hopes that I might "help her." Her adult head with perfect features rested on a body that had been severely twisted and foreshortened by the illness of her early childhood. Her thorax was hyperinflated; her rib cage rested atop her pelvis. A pediatric blood pressure cuff was too large for her withered arms. Her delicate fingers were scarcely thicker than the wire of coat hangers. She was paraplegic.

I hardly knew where to begin. She had high blood pressure and severe emphysema and psoriasis and extreme kyphoscoliosis. Her heart was massively enlarged. She had severe pulmonary hypertension.

At the end of our first visit I had compiled a page-long list of problems but no cohesive idea how I might help my new patient. I would need a second visit to complete my examination. Before she departed her mother opened her billfold to show me a faded black and white picture of a lovely blonde little girl taken weeks before her health had been smashed.

Mary Ruth's home pharmacy included diuretics, potassium supplements, antihypertensives, mucolytics, bronchodilators, and antibiotics. Her parents spotted potential problems early and managed her home therapy diligently and delicately. Bronchial infection posed a frequent hazard to her health. Because of early and unpleasant experiences in hospitals, she dreaded the thought of admission to any health care facility.

When Mary Ruth entered the waiting room of my office, other patients deflected their gaze only to later sneak looks at this diminutive, chair-bound lady. Several times I encountered her in shopping malls and cafeterias to which her parents frequently took her. Neither in my office waiting room nor in other public places did she seem self-conscious or afraid in any way.

On each visit I half-measured, half-estimated her blood pressure and listened to her lungs, which frequently exhibited wheezes or rales. Sometimes her feet and ankles were swollen. After the initial visit Mary Ruth detailed her symptoms while her mother or father sat quietly. We reviewed her many medications, sometimes altering a dose. She would review her activities. Her wisp-like fingers created delicate needlework. Her CB radio was easier to manipulate and allowed conversations with truckers and other acquaintances in her larger neighborhood.

Mary Ruth's health hovered always at the edge of chaos. I learned early that chest x-rays were of little value because most of her thorax was occupied by her gigantic heart. Empiricism ruled in the selection of types and doses of medications in combating frequent pulmonary infections. Mary Ruth and her parents addressed each crisis calmly. I never saw panic.

Over the years the hair of all of us either grayed or thinned. Her parents moved into their 80s; their gaits slowed and they fought their individual health problems. Each worried what would become of Mary Ruth after they had died. Mary Ruth grieved as she saw the health of her beloved parents fade. They continued to devote their dwindling strength to her care.

Her mother died first. Mary Ruth and her father moved into an apartment, where a visiting nurse supplemented his continued ministrations to his daughter.

Mary Ruth's breathing deteriorated. Remarkably, in her childhood years she had escaped placement in an iron lung. I do not know how she sustained her unaided breathing as long as she did. Finally, she required continuous oxygen therapy. She also required a motorized wheelchair.

Her father died. Her brother and two nieces shuffled work schedules to care for Mary Ruth in her single-room apartment. One morning Mary Ruth presented her plan to me. Her care was becoming increasingly complex, exceeding the time and energy that her devoted family could expend. It was time to enter a nursing home.

Sixty years after the polio outbreak in her Alabama community she visited my office once again.

"Here comes trouble. Your most troublesome patient is back," she announced.

She steered her motorized wheelchair into a now familiar examination room. Again I tried to obtain an accurate measure of her blood pressure. Her shallow breaths caused the slightest expansion of her chest. Her cardiac impulse extended across her entire chest.

We reviewed her medications. She spoke of friendships that she had established in the nursing home. When not visiting other patients or conversing in a community room, she liked to play blackjack and other games on a computer. She commented upon her graying hair and the aging that she noted in my thinning hair. She laughed easily and her eyes flashed, as they had repeatedly during each of 200 earlier visits. She returned to the van that would take her back to the nursing home.

She revered the memory of her parents. When bleak moments would occur, she reported that they had prayed together. After one heartbreaking setback, her mother had told her they would simply have to pray harder.

Sometimes I wonder if I have actually provided any care to Mary Ruth. I could never reverse any of the cruel damage to her body by that long-ago viral infection. Quite possibly, all of her medications could be discarded and there would be no difference in the functioning of any of her struggling organ systems. There were times when I urged hospitalization and she would decline. I did not feel anger or frustration, because I sensed a greater wisdom on the part of Mary Ruth and her parents. After all, they had repeatedly and successfully defied the pronouncements of medical experts since her illness began. They had nurtured a vibrant and loving spirit in a child whose body had been wrecked. I marvel at this miracle.

There are times when health care may consist of little more than a regular, hospitable conversation in which the mystery of life and the appalling consequences of disease are but background fixtures while two people review the day and prepare for another.

The vaccines, first injectable, now oral, removed the scourge of polio from the ken of all but its older victims and some of their surviving parents and friends. Occasionally, I see an atrophied leg or limp from an earlier infection. I have seen the depression that results when polio-afflicted limbs suddenly weaken further in later life. Polio casts long and terrible shadows.

Mary Ruth continues to teach me about patience and grace.

A LETTER FROM
THE GRAVE

Heroism takes many forms. Many heroes and heroines die or retire from the scene of their noble deeds with no special event, statue, or plaque to commemorate their special accomplishments. School teachers who sustain high professional standards despite difficult and discouraging surroundings belong to this pantheon. Somehow, these teachers never surrender the belief that they can raise the educational levels of their charges despite impoverished environments, poor community support, and limited aspirations of students and their parents. These educators are stubborn and creative, tireless, and endlessly patient with an unflagging commitment to a better world through humane education. James and Fannie Mathison were such a pair.

They had met during their teacher training. James had been hired to teach and coach in the high school of the small coal-mining community even before he had completed his college studies. He needed the money, and the school board had no certified teachers to fill the faculty vacancies. For a while he taught and commuted to a nearby college until he had earned his degree in history. Fannie told me that she knew at their first meeting that she would marry James. Marriage followed their graduation, and they settled in the community in which James already worked. Fannie began a career that was to span 50 years as an elementary school teacher.

James taught history and civics and coached the high school football team. A large and kind man, he read avidly, spoke with passion of the needs of public education, and voted a straight Democratic ticket. At mid-career he became school principal, a position he would hold until retirement.

"Didn't you ever get discouraged?" I asked one time, as he discussed the ongoing poverty and unemployment in his community.

"They are good people," he said. He would make certain that the children of these good people would have educational advantages and insights that their parents had lacked.

When the only physician in his community retired, James drove the 50 miles to my office for treatment of his hypertension and worsening osteoarthritis. He appeared always in a suit and tie. For a while after he retired, he and his wife, also now retired, considered relocation to a retirement community in the city in which they had attended college. His wife did not drive; James worried about what would happen to her should he become disabled or die.

At age 75 James almost died from cholangitis. Two years later a myocardial infarction claimed his life.

Fannie remained composed but grieved deeply. The couple had no children. Always, she maintained a regal bearing. Her tall, slender frame was perfectly postured, her gray hair precisely braided and wound into a tight bun. Like her husband she wore a conservatively tailored suit for each office appointment. Her blue eyes never flinched. She spoke precise English, with no east Tennessee inflection. Her carriage was so commanding that I could not imagine any student ever daring to breach the code of conduct in one of her classrooms.

Fannie suffered from hypertension and soon after James' death experienced her first episode of congestive heart failure. She chose to remain in their home rather than move to a retirement home. The mines and most other businesses in her home community had failed, but this was still her hometown. A niece in a distant city was her only relative.

As her health declined and episodes of heart failure became more frequent and protracted, Fannie became homebound. Former students chauffeured her to medical appointments and to the hairdresser, and they took her out to lunch each week. When illness further restricted Fannie's activity, alumni of her grade school made sure she had a hot meal daily and a warm-up meal available in her refrigerator. The love and respect of her companions for their teacher never flagged.

Fannie came close to death during a particularly severe episode of congestive failure that necessitated her final hospitalization. Her recovery was incomplete. We discussed the possibility of moving to a nursing home. There was no long-term care facility in her home community. She insisted upon returning home where, with the aid of a visiting nurse and ongoing support of her former students, she hoped to remain in her own space. Before leaving the hospital in the company of two of her former students, she told me that she could see no point in any future hospitalization.

Visiting nurses reported their assessments of Fannie to me regularly. Home oxygen therapy and diuretics maintained a reasonable level of comfort for her.

One morning the police called from her hometown to inform me of her death and to ask if I would sign her death certificate. She was 82. There was no one to whom I could express sympathy. My nurse and I were saddened as we returned to the day's patients.

Several weeks later, in the middle of a busy morning, the postman brought a registered bulky brown envelope to me. Inside, I found a note from the attorney who had handled Fannie's estate. The lawyer wrote that she had been instructed to transmit the enclosed envelope to me.

The envelope was addressed in Fannie's hand: "Please give this, unopened, to Dr. Clifton Cleaveland, Chattanooga, Tennessee."

Inside was a silver ring taped to this note:

Dear Dr. Cleaveland,

This is my engagement ring. Because you knew of the close bond between James and me—because you were with us during the worst times of our lives—and because you supported us through these times with your professional skill and understanding friendship, I want you to have this ring.

It is my wish that someone dear to you may wear it with as much love as I did for more than 50 years.

Sincerely,

Fannie

My wife wears the Mathison ring.

A SECOND LETTER

Each time Bill entered my office, the atmosphere became electric. He never engaged in casual conversation; rather, his every question or comment was precise and focused. I found myself sitting expectantly at the edge of my chair with my mind revved up to deal with Bill's inquiries. The oral portion of my medical board examinations required no more mental effort than these visits, in which Bill sought ever more detailed insights into his symptoms.

Bill was intense in all of his endeavors. He expected perfection from himself as well as from all who worked with him in his large engineering firm. A coworker described him as extremely demanding but never angry as he managed complex projects. Bill was divorced and stated that he could well understand how difficult it would be for any woman to live with him. His visits to my office extended over two decades, yet even after this interval he remained an enigma for me.

Bill's wiry athletic build and obsessive attention to diet and exercise belied severe coronary atherosclerosis. In his early 40s, anginal symptoms prompted his first coronary angiogram, which led in turn to multivessel coronary artery bypass. He blamed himself for this illness, although he had never been careless with his health. Profound depression complicated and prolonged his recovery. He was unable to return to work for many weeks, but once on the job he regained his preoperative drive.

Bill sought restoration of his health through a sabbatical at the Pritikin Institute. He returned to Chattanooga thinner than ever and worked more intensively at exercise and a vegetarian diet. During office visits he complained of daily, severe, throbbing headaches. He alluded to complex psychological stresses, which he declined to discuss. He rejected all recommendations for psychiatric consultation. Although I was his primary physician, he effectively designated much of his history off limits.

Several years later angina pectoris recurred and Bill required a second open-heart procedure. Once again deep depression impaired his recovery. His daily headaches intensified. Slowly and painfully he achieved a recovery sufficient to allow his return to work. He seemed insulted when I proposed that he reduce his responsibilities on the job. He intensified his exercise routine, which included early morning walks with his dog and intervals of intense training on his treadmill.

For a time Bill found happiness, meeting and subsequently marrying a lady in whose presence he appeared relaxed, and his smiles were less sardonic. In his wife's company he renewed a deep interest in classical music.

His daily workouts required multiple sublingual doses of nitroglycerin for completion. Nonetheless, he did not reduce the length or the intensity of any exercise program. Yet a third bypass, this using the last of available venous conduits, was performed. This time, with added intensive loving care by his wife, he had much less postoperative depression.

Although he initially improved to the point of sustained, brisk walking, Bill had daily attacks of angina pectoris. Typically, he used one or two nitroglycerin tablets each time he walked. Each contact with him, whether in my office or at a concert, remained spirited and intense. On one visit this most guarded of patients told me he had initiated visits to a psychiatrist. He spoke obliquely of complex problems that would appall me if I but knew the details. He had instructed his psychiatrist to report no information to me. Although he reported a sense of relief, he held out little prospect that psychotherapy would relieve his sorrows.

With no precipitating injury, Bill developed sciatica in his right leg. Rest and analgesics provided no relief. An MRI documented a herniated disc, and neurosurgery was performed without incident. The sciatic pain did not decrease. Electromyographic studies showed slight denervation in the distribution of the right sciatic nerve. Only when supine could Bill achieve any relief from the harassing pain. The best efforts of a sophisticated pain management clinic likewise failed to give comfort. His morose state equaled that which followed the first two coronary bypasses.

I had not seen Bill for several weeks when the police called. In a brief interval, while his wife was away from their home, Bill fatally shot himself. A few days later I received this note:

Dear Clifton,

Thank you so much for the past 20 years of help. I could not have gotten better. You are a great doctor and a wonderful person. And, hey, I didn't die of a heart attack.

Bill

This man of sustained sorrows to which he granted no access fought despair for 20 years. I could only guess at causes of the miseries that probably played a crucial role in provoking his heart disease and vascular headaches. Each day required a type of courage as he sought to move away from the despondency which was finally to wear him down.

I felt profoundly sad as I read and reread Bill's note. If only I could have found some means of entry into his troubles or some way to exploit the humor which showed even in his final note. I finally had a sense that Bill and I had each maintained separate medical files of his health and illnesses. We formulated separate expectations and prognoses. My friend chose to maintain a professional distance which I could never bridge. If only, if only.

JOKER WILD

The naked young woman screamed as she looked to the top of the waterfall that cascaded into the pool where she and her boyfriend splashed. A tall mound of brilliant orange suds hung momentarily at the crest of the falls before toppling onto the couple below. Neither could completely scrub the orange dye from their skin before reporting to work the next morning. Lamar, the jokester, was at it again.

Lamar worked in an automotive parts store and garage owned by his brother. The tie-dyed couple worked in the same business: she behind a desk, he in a tire-changing bay. Repeatedly the two left work early, each with a different excuse, each in a personal vehicle. Work piled up on the staff left behind. Lamar was dispatched one summer afternoon to follow the young man when he once again begged off work, complaining of a backache. A short distance from the store the couple united and drove in the man's pickup truck to a trailhead on Signal Mountain. The path led to a secluded pool at the base of a 20-foot high waterfall. There the couple shed their clothes to frolic in the cool blue water.

When informed of these observations, Lamar's brother wanted to fire, or at least severely reprimand, the swimmers. Lamar put forth an alternative plan to which his brother acquiesced. Lamar acquired a gallon of orange dye and a ten-gallon bucket of an industrial soap known for its sudsing quality. When next his coworkers set out for their mountain rendezvous, Lamar and his brother shadowed them. The couple hastened down the trail and shed their clothes on the flat boulders at water's edge before jumping into the pool.

The two men stealthily set about their work. Into the swirling white water upstream the men poured first the soap and then the dye from their perch on an overhanging rock.

"It was great, doc. You should have seen it," said Lamar.

The orange glacier rose and moved downstream, gathering at the crest of the falls before plopping like some giant meringue upon the screaming pair below.

Lamar reported that the young lovers maintained nearly perfect attendance records at work thereafter.

Another young worker in the garage repeatedly ceased his tasks to go to the single-seater men's toilet. After locking the door, he typically remained in the bathroom for 20 or more minutes. He carried lurid magazines into the cubicle. Repeated suggestions that he limit his excretory time were ignored.

Tired of his coworker's indolence Lamar rigged, one evening after work, a rubber hose, connecting it at one end to a powerful air compressor. The other end of the hose was concealed in the drainage pipe from the toilet.

The next morning the worker began his first toilet break. Lamar waited for a few minutes before activating the air compressor.

"God almighty!" The cry came from the john as the door burst open and the occupant leapt outside, pulling up his jeans in the same motion. A geyser of water rose from the toilet. Stares were exchanged; there were mutterings. The man recently dislodged from the toilet seat groused about unfair treatment. His subsequent visits to the toilet were shorter and less frequent.

Lamar was tall and rangy with a military style crew cut. When he initiated his drawled speech, he raised his eyebrows and his words came with a smile. He paused always before replying to an inquiry as if reviewing the logic of his response. He was accustomed to very hard work. For years he cleared forested and boulder-strewn land for new home sites. In his 40s, work which he previously tolerated with ease caused dyspnea and palpitations. He came to my office for the first time.

His heart was enlarged. His pulse was rapid and he had frequent premature heartbeats. An echocardiogram and a subsequent cardiac catheterization documented congestive cardiomyopathy and significant mitral valve incompetence. With medication his symptoms diminished. Although he tried for weeks to sustain the pace and demands of his land-clearing enterprise, his health would not cooperate, and he was forced to shut down his company.

Once, while he worked to clear a particularly steep and rocky lot, the developer for the proposed subdivision arrived in his truck. As he wandered over the rough terrain, he cursed Lamar and his two coworkers repeatedly. The following morning, when the developer entered his truck, he could not turn the steering wheel because of a fine coating of black cup grease that had been applied lightly to the circumference.

Even the reduced work load at his brother's auto parts store proved taxing for Lamar's heart. His brother recognized Lamar's limitations and urged that he work less hard and go home mid-afternoon. Lamar persisted in putting in a full day of effort. Larger doses of medication were needed to forestall arrhythmia and congestive heart failure. At each visit Lamar wanted the facts of his case presented in a straightforward manner. When I mentioned the possibility that he might need to take a disability retirement, he dismissed the idea.

Lamar was married with two teenaged children. His home, before which he had placed a totem pole, was a magnet for all the children in the neighborhood. When not restoring old motorcycles, he taught the children how to use common tools to fix things. I visited his home late one afternoon. As I pulled into his driveway, Lamar waved from his front stoop where he sat surrounded by several children from the neighborhood. Besides useful information, he dispensed candy and, from time to time, ice cream.

A neighbor owned a three-wheeled, all-terrain vehicle with large rear tires. At any hour the youth fired up his noisy vehicle, driving across front and back lawns of his neighbors. Their complaints failed to reform his thoughtlessness. When Lamar found tracks from the three-wheeler across the torn corner of his vegetable garden, he had had enough.

With the guile of a saboteur, Lamar crept into the shed where the monster machine was kept. The owner was away for the weekend. Lamar removed each of the large rear wheels, filling each half full of quick-setting cement. When replaced on the rear axle, the tires appeared normally inflated. Lamar was working in his yard the next time his neighbor fired up his tricycle. He turned quickly, just in time to see the rider trying to control his machine on a zigzag course that ended in a large bush at the foot of his driveway.

Lamar recounted his prankish vendettas with relish. He spoke with equal delight of his children. He was confident of their strength and knew that they would provide comfort and support to his wife should his health collapse.

Lamar's health unraveled. His mitral valve gave way. Urgent open heart surgery was his only hope. He died soon after valve replacement.

At the wake Lamar rested in the open casket clad in a favorite plaid shirt and khaki pants. The room was filled with flowers. The card on one read in a childish print: "To the ice cream man from his gang."

His pastor told the crowded congregation how this man of modest means had quietly provided funds over the years to buy shoes for needy children in his mountain neighborhood.

Lamar's wife and children delivered to my house a large green plant from the funeral. They grieved. Lamar had discussed carefully with each of them how they would make it once he was gone, and they did.

Lamar's brother had the most difficult time dealing with the loss. He missed the goodness, the jests, and the hard work that his brother personified. One day, after he recounted yet another of Lamar's exploits, the brother said, "That Lamar, he was a pistol."

DELLA'S ARM

"You'll think I'm crazy. Sometimes in the middle of the night I get up and hold her hand. All I do is sit there and cry. I miss her so much. I don't know how I'll make it."

Miller sat slumped slightly forward, looking unblinkingly at nothing in particular. He spoke in a monotone of Della, who had been dead these many months.

The first trouble with Della's arm appeared in her early teen years. A minor fall, as she remembered, fractured her right humerus near the shoulder. X-rays suggested something else, possibly a tumor at the fracture site. This prompted a biopsy by an orthopedic surgeon. The diagnosis was fibrous dysplasia. Additional x-rays showed similar lesions in the right side of her bony pelvis and right femur.

Because the fracture of her humerus did not heal, various authorities rendered an opinion as to the most preferred therapy. Eventually surgery was undertaken, and the interior of the humerus was cleaned of its abnormal fibrotic material. Steel rods were inserted in hopes that normal bone might form around this scaffolding.

A second minor fall caused a fresh break.

Experts in another city recommended a course of radiation to her right arm, pelvis, and femur. Another break of the right humerus required a bone graft.

Della recalled amputation being first mentioned as a possible therapy when she turned 20. The medical opinions that she and her family sought in cities throughout the Southeast were contradictory. Despite constant pain and the uncertainty of what lay ahead, Della seemed undaunted and gave little outward sign to her friends of any abiding burden of illness.

At 25 she met Miller, and soon thereafter they married. He treasured his fair-skinned, blonde bride, a lady of charm, sparkle, and ready wit.

More battles to save the arm ensued. Pain was constant. The muscles of her right arm withered. Finally, at age 35, it happened. A rounded, firm mass rapidly grew near Della's right shoulder. X-rays suggested, and biopsies confirmed, a fibrosarcoma. There was no option to surgery. Right arm, right scapula, and all regional lymph nodes were removed. There seemed to be no extension of the dreaded cancer beyond the right arm. She received additional radiation therapy.

A year later Della shopped for a new arm. She read every available article that described prostheses. Miller shared her quest for the perfect artificial arm. They located a company in another city where, after extensive measurements, an arm was fashioned.

And what an arm! From a distance of a few feet, in its slightly flexed posture, her right arm appeared to be a real part of her. Touch revealed its synthetic nature. Coloration of the new limb matched her own honey-colored skin, with a scattering of tan freckles. The creases over the knuckles of the slightly flexed fingers were perfect. Her fingernails glistened with transparent polish and matched those of her left hand exactly. Gentle ridges of extensor tendons and delicate superficial veins decorated the dorsum of her new hand. A fortune teller could have read her future in the lines of the palm. A new dimension was added to the concept of wearable art.

She preferred long-sleeved blouses. Sometimes she might roll up the cuff a turn or two. Once I saw her carry a jacket, neatly folded, across her right forearm.

Life seemed stable. Fortunately, the dysplastic areas of her right leg remained quiescent despite extensive, prior radiation therapy.

Della became my patient at that point. I recall a cheerful, neatly dressed, slender young woman. Miller accompanied her. They spoke to each other intermittently, sometimes to establish an historical point, sometimes to share a chuckle. Then and during subsequent visits our communication involved a three-sided conversation. Della exhibited her right arm with pride. Our shared concern was the monitoring for any recurrent or new malignancy.

When she was in her early 40s, she developed a cough. Chest x-ray showed ominous, enlarged lymph nodes about her trachea and bronchi. Surprisingly, a biopsy of one of the nodes showed sarcoidosis. Steroids quieted her worsening cough. After a few months her intrathoracic lymph nodes shrank to almost normal size. Miller had feared the worst; Della reassured him that she would quickly recover. She never exhibited fear, anger, or despair.

Two years later fresh nodules appeared in her lungs. This time the biopsy showed fibrosarcoma. Oncologists advised intravenous chemotherapy. Della's peripheral veins quickly proved inadequate for repeated infusions. An arteriovenous shunt placed in her left leg solved the problem of access for her medication. Her wit never flagged. It was Miller who sat quiet and fearful at each visit. Della was as matter-of-fact in her attitude as if she was simply bringing a kitchen appliance in for repair.

One Sunday afternoon my doorbell rang. As Miller and Della returned from a picnic in a nearby state park they decided to visit my wife and me. The masterpiece right arm extended from the short sleeve of her bright orange blouse. Certain people bring into any setting a sense that a party or a celebration is about to begin. Della was the chairman of this group. I could never recall a meeting with Della in any setting that I did not laugh repeatedly. This visit was no exception. Miller remained quiet, looking at his wife with wonder and a slight smile.

Chemotherapy brought a reprieve of a year. Then multiple tumor masses exploded into her lungs and throughout her body. Although pale and weak, her infectious good humor persisted undiminished. She resisted hospitalization, but finally there was no alternative. She could no longer eat. Her pain needed intravenous medication for relief.

As I entered her room I sensed she was dying. Both arms rested above the sheet. Even at the point of death she wanted the cherished false arm displayed. Her left arm, by contrast, was pale and wasted. Her wet and labored respirations faded. Earlier, Della had made it quite clear that there were to be no resuscitative efforts or placement in an intensive care unit. Miller, a nurse-friend, and I stood at her bedside. Miller held her true hand. And then her breathing stopped.

We reminisced at her bedside. I said a prayer. Her pastor arrived and read from the Book of Revelation.

Two days later at her funeral the minister spoke of her victory, of a little girl with a steadily worsening developmental defect, probably cast at conception's moment. He spoke of a grandfather to whom she attributed her courage. Her pastor reviewed the highlights of a full and happy life. He reminded us of the happiness she inspired in others.

The hearse pulled away from the church, and I returned to my office.

Miller came to the office a time or two. He worked harder than ever at his managerial job, trying to cope with his sorrow. In contrast to his wife's bravery, he feared a future of solitude.

Months later we sat in an examining room. Miller's mild hypertension remained under control. He spoke of holding his beloved's hand. Della had been buried without her prosthesis. This had been held back; possibly this very expensive device could be modified for someone else's use. The prosthesis had been carefully wrapped in a sheet and placed in the bottom drawer of an armoire.

In the sorrow of a sleepless and tear-choked night, Miller arose from his bed. Seated on the floor, he opened the bottom drawer, searched out the fingers, and pulled Della's wrist and hand free of the linen so that he might clasp the hand and speak to her of the grief in his heart. Other nights followed in which he continued his monologues.

"You think I'm crazy, don't you?" he asked.

"Not at all, Miller. Not at all," I said.

Other patients tell me that, following the loss of spouses, they too speak to their absent loved ones. A retired kindergarten teacher cried at each visit following her husband's death. She felt incompetent to manage any of the business aspects of her household. Her husband had balanced the checkbook, tracked expenses, completed the tax forms, and maintained the home and yard.

"I talk to his picture at night and tell him my problems," she said. If a fright awakened her at night, she turned on a bedside light next to his picture, which she left illuminated until dawn. She felt his presence and knew reassurance.

Another widow startled her grown children by telling of a nightly chat with their father, who had died six years earlier. They worried that she was losing her sanity and would soon need placement in a nursing home.

A patient who is quite rational spoke to me of the comfort that she felt when, after solitary suppers, she closed her eyes and spoke of the day's events. She imagined her husband once again seated in his favorite upholstered chair. She addressed him as "Honey."

Yet another widow, a lady in her 80s, alarmed a friend who accompanied her home following dinner at a restaurant. Upon opening her front door, the widow said loudly, "I'm home, Dear." Sensing her companion's surprise, the widow said, "It's a habit, I suppose, I'll never get over."

The memory of love can assume an almost visible presence. For Miller, the icon of his Della's arm served as a trigger for a rush of recollections. He had loved her for 25 years. He had been a cowarrior in the war against her cancer, the survivor of an all-out but ultimately losing effort. Both a beloved comrade and a battle had been lost. Emptiness and sorrow were joined with the exhaustion of a profound defeat. With time, Miller could recount events of their shared past without tears. He would laugh upon recalling a comedic moment. Eventually he moved to another city. I do not know the fate of Della's arm.

THE MAN WHO
COULD NOT DIE

As a boy in rural Troupe County, Georgia, he had seen a pack of rabid dogs tearing down the dirt road as he stood behind his plow. They were too far away to sense him. He stood motionless, lest they catch his movement and turn their crazed motion up the hill toward him in this furrowed field.

Once the boy had ridden in a wagon with his parents and some of his brothers and sisters to visit a neighbor's farm. The head of that house was dying from rabies. The boy caught a glimpse of the neighbor bound tightly to his bed frame, arching his back and making the most dreadful of sounds. He would never forget the shrieks. The door was quickly closed to shield the children.

The boll weevil and a collapsing farm economy drove the family into town, where his mother rented rooms to boarders. One tried to trim a bunion from his foot with a razor. A month later the man, a door-to-door salesman, lost his leg to the ensuing infection. He died soon thereafter.

The boy wanted to be like his uncle, a physician. A friend who had some money in the tight economic times of the early '20s offered to pay some of his college cost; an uncle promised aid as well. But he could not afford time away from his salaried job. Long hours at the pharmacy on the town square precluded completion even of high school. He hoped he might resume his studies someday.

The pharmacist recognized the boy's quickness and taught him to mix the flavorings, colorings, and potions that comprised much of the pharmacopeia. He became expert at deciphering the prescriptions regularly brought in by patients. One physician simply wrote "#1," "#2," or "#3" to specify a particular concoction for a troubled patient.

The lot of physicians was none too secure. In the second-floor space above the pharmacy, free rent was accorded three physicians in exchange for a monopoly on filling their prescriptions. Of the three doctors one was to die of tuberculosis, and another ran off with his nurse to Oklahoma never to return.

The doctors remained in their offices late on Friday and Saturday nights. When a fight broke out in the town's pool hall or when an accident or shooting occurred, the physicians raced to the scene. The first doctor there won the right to pick the patient. Sometimes the pharmacist's aide would be in tow, brought along to help carry the wounded and bashed back to the physician's office. After a melee, there might be two patients for the swiftest doctor. There was no emergency room in the small hospital, and only the near-dead would be taken there anyway. Sometimes the pharmacist's aide was permitted to finish the suturing or apply the bulky dressings if the physician was too tired or if he was called to other scenes of trauma. Sometimes a physician might be too inebriated to complete the work.

The boy was now a young man. He knew which physicians battled alcoholism and which used cocaine. As he shuttled from the pharmacy to the offices above, he heard more than he wanted to know of beatings, sorrows, and betrayals. He still wanted to be a doctor.

The young man was a good salesman, and an insurance manager hired him away from the pharmacy for $15 a week and chances for commissions to boot. He pounded the pavement in that mill town and other mill towns in west and north Georgia, selling policies and collecting 25-cent and 50-cent weekly premiums.

The man prospered and married, and soon fathered two children. He ate too much food, smoked too many cigars, and sometimes drank too much bourbon. He hired many new agents to sell insurance for the company, which he now managed. He was promoted to a larger office in a city 300 miles from his roots. At retirement time, health, which had been previously blemished only by recurring attacks of acute gout, deteriorated. An eyelid drooped. He had trouble swallowing. Eventually, the label of myasthenia gravis was attached to his symptoms. He did not care much for the medications, which caused diarrhea.

His pulse slowed, and he was dizzy. A pacemaker fixed this, but the gout worsened, further destabilizing joints already stressed by his 280 pounds.

At 75 his myasthenia forced him into a recliner. A neurologist advised azathioprine. For a while his muscles responded to the new medication. He could walk about his yard and sprinkle shrubbery with a hose.

He passed blood. A colon cancer was identified and removed.

He developed a red and spreading rash over his hands and forearms. Biopsy and culture diagnosed the fungus Cryptococcus; blood cultures yielded the organism as well. In the hospital he tolerated with difficulty weeks of antifungal medication. An internist, a cardiologist, an infectious disease specialist, a general surgeon, and a neurologist collaborated in his care. His children were called home; the whole family made plans for his funeral. He rallied and returned home to the recliner positioned by a favorite window through which he could survey his yard and follow the comings and goings on the street beyond.

He maintained contact with his country boyhood with a weekly trip to a nearby farmers' market, where he could drive by the individual stalls and speak to the farmers about their crops and how much a bushel of corn might be worth.

One day, while his wife was at the grocery store, he became so short of breath he felt he would die. He tapped the window pane with his cane until a neighbor could be attracted. An ambulance was called. He was admitted with a massive pulmonary embolus from which recovery was not expected.

He returned home. He had cataracts removed. His prostate required transurethral surgery. He developed a worsening skin rash. This time the diagnosis was bullous pemphigoid. When his grandchildren visited, his strength permitted hugs only. He spoke to them of olden times and relished their visits. Next to his family, he loved most the Atlanta Braves, whose every game he watched on television. He spoke of his hope that he would survive to see his team win a World Series.

At 86 years, one day his right foot hurt worse than ever before. Not even a dreaded gout attack caused such misery. His weight had been decreasing; he weighed less than 200 pounds for the first time in decades. Ultrasound studies showed no circulation in his right leg, and angiography demonstrated arteries beyond hope of bypass or repair. It would have to be an above-the-knee amputation, and he wanted to know how long before he could return home.

The preoperative chest x-ray showed lungs filled with a snow-storm of metastases, and there was a new mass in the left side of his ab-domen. Amputation was postponed.

It was time to go home, but first I had to fulfill a promise to tell him if ever he were in a hopeless and untreatable situation. We had dodged the question many times before when hope, which had been reduced to a spark, would glow and then flame when another illness had been defeated.

I entered his room, sat on his bed, and spoke of changes in his lungs for which there was no therapy. Comfort would be the goal. It was time to leave this hospital, and he would not need to return ever again. He belonged at home. He needed to be home.

Just then the dreaded quaver hit my voice, and I could go no fur-ther. I buried my face in the sagging skin where shoulder and neck met. I remember saying, "Thank you for taking care of me."

And my father, this man who had wanted to go to medical school and whose pride I felt in being a physician, put his arm about my shoulders and said, "It'll be okay, boy." From earliest memory I had been referred to as "boy."

He returned home by ambulance two days later.

My father's care by his internist and his subspecialty colleagues had been and remained masterful and compassionate. Always my father had run by me the latest recommendation, finding, or wrinkle in therapy.

My identities as son and physician were intertwined. I could not compartmentalize my two roles. The son sought optimistic answers and ached deeply when the news was bad. The physician ran mental scans of pertinent medical information when a fresh crisis arose. I struggled at times to deal with the competing tensions of my two identities. I came to see, however, that the expectations of love and the inquiries of science are not necessarily antithetical. The goals of both love and science can be congruent: freedom from suffering, sustenance of an independent life in cherished surroundings, freedom from fear. To the objectivity of science, love adds the dimensions of reasonableness and compassion.

My father lived for four more months, seldom able to leave his bed during the final weeks. Remarkably, my mother's health held as she kept this large man from toppling the final few feet.

On my last visit, a flight to his South Carolina home five days before his death, I could feel the giant mass in his belly as we bathed him. He spoke with greater effort. He recounted another of the stories from his almost-doctor days.

During the afternoon of my visit I saw one of the gentlest acts of compassion by a fellow professional. My father's dentist knew of his failing health. This good man made a home visit to check my father's dentures, which were now too loose to be functional. He sat at my father's bedside, shaping and pasting, until the dentures would hold in place and the final few meals could be enjoyed.

My father willed his body to a medical school. We celebrated the stories of his life at a memorial service.

EPILOGUE

"Betty," I spoke to the sleeping figure.

She stirred, rubbed her eyes and mumbled, "Is that you, Doc?"

"Yes. Your surgery is over," I told her.

"Praise Jesus. He ain't never let me down," she said.

These were the words of my patient, Betty Terry, as she awakened in the hospital's recovery room following a procedure that had demonstrated the cruel extent of a malignancy of her lower face. At that moment I was relieved that she had survived. It took me years to understand the true meaning of her words.

She worked as a cleaning lady on the medical ward of Erlanger Hospital long before such jobs were designated as environmental services. No matter how tired this woman might seem, she was always cheerful; her greetings to patients and staff were never perfunctory. Twenty years after her death, a retired nurse from that medical unit became teary as she described to me her own encounters with this lady of such gentle spirit.

One day, as I began my early morning rounds, Betty asked if I would be her doctor. I accepted her request immediately. She suffered from hypertension and worn-out joints. Mopping, sweeping, and emptying waste cans for eight hours each day had to be painful, but she never acknowledged it as she moved about with obvious great effort. Sometimes she came to my office, but more often she sought advice or a brief exam of an ailing part as we met during our work at the hospital.

She stopped me one morning to ask me to check a nodule on her lower jaw. This was the beginning of a neoplasm that would soon take her life. Surgery was extensive, resulting in the loss of her left mandible and much of the soft tissue of her neck. Extensive tumor remained. It was following this intervention that she regained consciousness in the recovery room in my presence.

Radiation failed to check the rapid advance of the cancer. Her wound never healed and remained a site of recurrent drainage and infection. Jane Plumlee, my nurse for all these years, accompanied me on visits to Betty's apartment as we did what we could to clean the gaping hole in her upper neck and lessen her suffering. Her smile and warmth of welcome remained intact, just as they had in her work. Her grown children rotated a continuous presence at her bedside.

From Betty Terry I began to comprehend the fallacy in the notion that as a physician I "take a history." Rather, I take in my patient's story, sometimes sequentially, sometimes in scattered, almost random segments. This story, if honored with time and privacy, defines an immediate illness or problem not as some isolated calamity but as part of a continuity of experience. This history speaks to the dreams and fears, regrets and joys of a unique person.

This story defines relationships and identifies the patient's physical and spiritual home. The physical home is the deeply personal space imbued with the artifacts, icons, and memories that have become as inseparable from the individual as the shell would be for a box turtle. The spiritual home is the aggregate of all the experiences, daydreams, reflections, and deepest searchings that define us as individuals. Sick or injured, we long to repair to both.

Betty Terry's story was like a delicate mosaic of which I was shown a tile or two at a time. Much remained unstated but was no less evident in relating what this lady cherished. From the outset I knew that her family was her pride and source of delight. When her health began to crumble, she was insistent in seeking the earliest possible dismissal from the hospital to return to her home where her family could surround her. This modest and sparsely furnished space was impeccably clean. Her bedclothes were bleached and freshly pressed. This was her nest, her refuge, the center of innumerable comings and goings of the children and friends whom she loved.

In the same way that Betty Terry and her children welcomed me into her home, I had been welcomed into the story of her life. As I learned of her values and traditions, I could customize medical science to meet her particular needs. I could see the nuances of questions that sought so much more than reassurance.

During my formal training, a medical history was presented as a physician-directed interrogation bounded by the time restraints of an appointment or rounding schedule. The detailed and immediate facts of an illness are, of course, vital to the solving of a medical problem, but this is only one aspect of what we must garner if care is to be personal and respectful. People are no more generic than their myriad illnesses in their countless presentations.

When, as in Betty Terry's case, I can visit a patient over time, I realize that a medical history never ends. Facts, insights, passions, and revisions constantly expand and reshape the story, its narrator as well as its listener.

I, the physician, was no passive listener to Betty Terry or my other patients and teachers. She and they deepened my comprehension of love and loyalty, humor and sacrifice, both in their lives as well as my own. Through their experiences I could begin to plumb my own strengths and limitations.

In understanding the strength and comfort derived by my patients and teachers from their varied religious faiths, I came to see God not limited to narrow sectarian restraints or formal worship but ever-present and available to each of us in the uniqueness of our lives. This spiritual dialogue is just as likely to find expression in imaginative literature, a melodic refrain, or a view over quiet water at dusk as from a structured, religious observance. The interfaces of the spiritual with the lives of my patients and my teachers have been numerous and continuing. I believe it was gratitude for this continuity that Betty Terry expressed as she awakened.

The stories to which I have been privy speak of individual journeys toward uncertain destinations. Some of these voyages are over, some are still under way. These journeys have taught me to be more aware of my own. The sacred space is where our journeys coincide.

ABOUT THE AUTHOR

Clif Cleaveland, MD, MACP, grew up in LaGrange, Georgia, and Columbia, South Carolina. Following graduation from Duke University he attended Oxford University as a Rhodes scholar, receiving a master of arts degree in animal physiology. He earned his medical degree from Johns Hopkins University before serving his internship and medical residency at Vanderbilt University Hospital. After Army service at Fort Knox and a fellowship in clinical pharmacology at Vanderbilt, he began medical practice in Chattanooga, Tennessee. He and his wife, Ruzha, have four children and two grandchildren.